Pediatric Triage Guidelines

Pediatric Triage Guidelines

Kathleen A. Murphy, MSN, RN, CEN

Nursing Education Council

Emergency Department

The Children's Hospital of Philadelphia

Philadelphia, Pennsylvania

Executive Director

Pediatric Educators, Inc.

West Chester, Pennsylvania

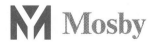

St. Louis Baltimore Boston Carlsbad Chicago Naples New York Philadelphia Portland
London Madrid Mexico City Singapore Sydney Tokyo Toronto Wiesbaden

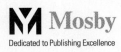

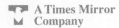

Vice President and Publisher: Nancy L. Coon
Senior Editor: Sally Schrefer
Associate Developmental Editor: Michele D. Hayden
Project Manager: Dana Peick
Senior Production Editor: Stavra Demetrulias
Design Coordinator: Amy Buxton
Manufacturing Manager: David Graybill

Printed in the United States of America
Composition by Black Dot Group
Printing/binding by R.R. Donnelly

Mosby-Year Book, Inc.
11830 Westline Industrial Drive
St. Louis, Missouri 63146

0-8151-7333-4

96 97 98 99 00 / 9 8 7 6 5 4 3 2 1

Consultants

editorial
Steven M. Selbst, MD
Director, Emergency Department
The Children's Hospital of Philadelphia;
Associate Professor of Pediatrics
University of Pennsylvania School of Medicine
Philadelphia, Pennsylvania

nursing
Cathleen Longo, MSN, RN, CEN, CCRN
Staff Nurse, Emergency Department
The Children's Hospital of Philadelphia;
Pediatric Nursing Faculty Instructor
University of Pennsylvania School of Nursing
Philadelphia, Pennsylvania

Contributors

Christine Heller, BSN, RN
Director of Supply, Processing, & Distribution
The Children's Hospital of Philadelphia
Philadelphia, Pennsylvania

Cathy Knox-Fisher, MSN, RN
Mental Health Clinical Nurse Specialist
The Children's Hospital of Philadelphia
Philadelphia, Pennsylvania

Zibigniew Kornecki, BSN, RN, CEN
Staff Nurse, Emergency Department
The Children's Hospital of Philadelphia
Philadelphia, Pennsylvania

Monica Liebman, MSN, RN
Trauma Clinical Nurse Specialist
The Children's Hospital of Philadelphia
Philadelphia, Pennsylvania

Patricia D. Minges, RN, CEN
Staff Nurse, Emergency Department
The Children's Hospital of Philadelphia
Philadelphia, Pennsylvania

Mary A. Verderame, BSN, RN, CEN, CPN
Staff Nurse, Emergency Department
The Children's Hospital of Philadelphia
Philadelphia, Pennsylvania

Reviewers

Ann Marie Capelli Anderson, RN
  Clinical Research Associate
  Shriners Hospital for Crippled
    Children
  St. Louis, Missouri

Jane Barnsteiner, PhD, RN, FAAN
  Director of Nursing Practice &
    Research
  The Children's Hospital of Philadelphia
  Philadelphia, Pennsylvania

Robin Gallay Fremer, MSN, RN
  Clinical Associate
  Department of Family and Community
  Ohio State University
    College of Nursing
  Columbus, Ohio

Fred M. Henretig, MD
  Attending Physician,
    Emergency Department
  The Children's Hospital of Philadelphia;
  Medical Director
  Poison Control Center
  Philadelphia, Pennsylvania

Monica Liebman, MSN, RN
  Trauma Clinical Nurse Specialist
  The Children's Hospital of
    Philadelphia;
  Philadelphia, Pennsylvania

Cathleen Longo, MSN, RN, CCRN, CEN
  Staff Nurse, Emergency Department
  The Children's Hospital of Philadelphia;
  Pediatric Nursing Faculty Instructor
  University of Pennsylvania
    School of Nursing
  Philadelphia, Pennsylvania

Stephen Ludwig, MD
  Associate Chair for Medical Education
  The Children's Hospital of Philadelphia;
  Professor of Pediatrics
  University of Pennsylvania
    School of Medicine
  Philadelphia, Pennsylvania

Steven M. Selbst, MD
  Director, Emergency Department
  The Children's Hospital of Philadelphia;
  Associate Professor of Pediatrics
  University of Pennsylvania
    School of Medicine
  Philadelphia, Pennsylvania

Rob Sheridan, MD
  Assistant Chief of Staff
  Shriners Hospital for Crippled Children
  Burn Institute
  Boston, Massachusetts

Janet F. Sullivan, PhD, RN, CPNP
  Clinical Associate Professor of Nursing
  Department of Parent-Child Health
    Nursing
  State University of New York
    at Stony Brook
  Stony Brook, New York

Ann Summers, MS, RN, CRNP
  Pediatric Nurse Practitioner
  York, Pennsylvania

Ronald Tompkins, MD, ScD
  Chief of Staff
  Shriners Hospital for Crippled
    Children
  Burn Institute
  Boston, Massachusetts

Elizabeth Warmke, MS, RN
  Pediatric/PICU Clinical Nurse
    Specialist
  Christ Hospital and Medical Center
  Oak Lawn, Illinois

Foreword

Triage is a word that is derived from the French. Its literal meaning is to divide in three parts or to sort. The term was originally used on the battlefields of Europe in order to medically sort casualties into groups: those who cannot be expected to survive, those who will recover without treatment and those who require immediate treatment in order to survive. The original meaning of the term and its application have undergone change as have other medical terms. Triage still means sorting but instead of the battlefield it is most often used in modern emergency medical care in the hospital and the pre-hospital setting. The spirit of the original definition was to apply the appropriate resources to the appropriate population of injured patients. This spirit has been maintained in the crowd of the busy urban emergency setting where we also seek to apply our resources to the best outcome.

The roots of this book and the modern pediatric emergency medicine triage process began at the Children's Hospital of Philadelphia in 1975. It was here that we began an effort to improve pediatric emergency services in our own setting and across the United States. Our emergency department had moved from an older site to a new hospital and the patient census had increased from 25,000 patient visits per year to what would become more than 70,000 visits. In some ways it did feel like a battlefield scene. We tried many combinations and permutations to solve our patient flow problems but settled on a triage strategy as a way of classifying patients and making sure no severely ill or injured child was waiting in the corner of our overcrowded waiting room. Over the succeeding years, we quickly learned many lessons about triage and about the qualities that it took to do the job correctly and efficiently.

The first thing that was done was to codify the rules and regulations of triage in a manual far more crude than the book that follows. Secondly, we realized that effective triage required more than knowledge than could be placed on sheets of paper. We found that it took experience and a sixth sense to know who was sick and who was not. This was demonstrated most clearly when we substituted our first triage officers, our pediatric residents, with our most senior nurses. The nurses, many of whom were parents themselves, were far more skilled in getting the right patient to the right place at the ED. Finally, we learned that it was not just a matter of knowledge and experience, but an ability to meet and work with the public in a unique human interaction setting. Many of our first nurses became burned-out as we would assign them to triage for a full eight or twelve hour shift. This was a task too great for any individual no matter how calm and balanced they were. The interpersonal stresses were simply too great. So, again we learned, and modified our practice.

So, the practice has been modified and modified again. It has been honed to a fine practice art in itself as it is described in the many instructive sections that follow. Kathleen Murphy has written an excellent book. With her colleagues she presents the ultimate in Pediatric Triage Guidelines. It is complete, thorough, and well documented. Like the work done on the battlefields of France, I know it will save lives, soothe the emotions of frightened parents, and allow us to use our scarce medical resources most wisely. I salute the author, her collaborators, and the many colleagues and patients that taught us along the way.

Stephen Ludwig, MD
Associate Chair for Medical Education
The Children's Hospital of Philadelphia;
Professor of Pediatrics
University of Pennsylvania School of Medicine
Philadelphia, Pennsylvania

Preface

This book was developed in response to the need for comprehensive pediatric triage protocols and guidelines. The intent of the book is to assist health care providers in understanding and implementing a triage system that provides safe and efficient care to the pediatric population.

The material in this book was designed for use by registered nurses, advanced practice nurses, school nurses, pre-hospital care providers, and physicians in a formalized Emergency Department or community setting. The book is user friendly and can be a resource for any health care professional who cares for children in the acute, nonacute, or chronic care environment.

Pediatric Triage Guidelines contains 142 triage protocols, each presented on two facing pages for ease of use. A complete listing of presenting symptoms and interventions for the health care provider are included for each protocol, and the four triage categories are clearly delineated for quick decision making and intervention. The book also includes the latest JCAHO requirements for triage competency behaviors to ensure quality improvement and safe practice standards.

Additional reference information is included in sections I, II, and III of the book and in the Appendices, to make this the most comprehensive book available on pediatric triage.

Acknowledgements

Many of my professional colleagues and friends at the Children's Hospital of Philadelphia made suggestions and comments that greatly improved the character and quality of this book. I am grateful for their comments, encouragement, and support. I am also grateful to those leaders in our profession who have developed the groundwork and theoretical concepts that made this triage guide possible.

I would like to express my sincere thanks to Jane Barnsteiner, PhD, RN; Carole Burdge, MSN, RN; Paula Levine, MA, RN; Steven M. Selbst, MD; Stephen Ludwig, MD; and the dedicated medical and nursing staff in the Emergency Department at the Children's Hospital of Philadelphia for their honorable contributions and guidance during the development of this book. I would also like to express my heartfelt gratitude to my family, Gary, Andrew, Mom, and Dad, for their patience, love and enduring support over the past years.

Again, many thanks.
Kathleen A. Murphy

Contents

SECTION IV: Pediatric Triage Protocols

SECTION V: APPENDICES

Pediatric Triage Guidelines

Section I

Introduction to Pediatric Triage

How To Use the Triage Guidelines

Pediatric Triage Guidelines is a reference book designed for health care providers to standardize and prioritize patient care according to the child's severity of illness. The severity of illness is determined by compiling and evaluating the following: the child's subjective complaints, presenting signs and symptoms, physical assessment parameters, and vital signs. This book is designed with specific triage protocols to assist in "classifying" the child according to the severity of illness. The child's classification can fall into one of four categories: Critical, Acute, Urgent, or Nonurgent.

Triage Classification of Acuity

CLASS I: CRITICAL

Pediatric patients who present with life- or limb-threatening illnesses or injuries requiring emergency medical and nursing intervention are classified as critical. These patients are in *immediate* need of advanced emergency care that requires stabilization or resuscitation at a designated trauma center or emergency department (ED).

CLASS II: ACUTE

Pediatric patients who present with significant alterations in their physical or mental health that could potentially become life or limb threatening are classified as acute. These patients require medical and nursing intervention *as soon as possible* at an ED.

CLASS III: URGENT

Pediatric patients who present with significant physical or mental health problems that are not life or limb threatening are classified as urgent. These patients will receive appropriate medical and nursing interventions in *a timely fashion* at either their primary pediatrician's office, an urgent care center, or an ED.

CLASS IV: NONURGENT

Pediatric patients who present with stable physical or mental health problems are classified as nonurgent. These patients are at no immediate risk for loss of life or limb and may receive care at either their primary care physician's office or at a medical clinic *when convenient*.

Important: The patient's condition and triage classification may change at any time after the initial evaluation, where there is often a need for registered nurse (RN) or physician reassessment. Address any concerns related to the patient's triage classification with the health care provider who made the initial evaluation.

Goals of Pediatric Triage

The overall goals of triage are multifaceted. Triage provides a general but brief evaluation of *all* incoming patients to the ED. This evaluation is accomplished through a concise primary and secondary survey. This survey is necessary to determine which patients are in need of immediate care and which patients can wait for delayed care without adverse outcomes. A comprehensive triage system also increases the safety and efficiency of patient care by regulating the flow of patients through the ED. In addition, an efficient triage system decreases the congestion in the emergency treatment areas and aids the delivery of appropriate care in an orderly and timely fashion. The expeditious care and treatment of all patients ultimately allows for a more rapid, safer delivery of services to those in need of emergent medical and nursing intervention.

Pediatric Triage Objectives

The primary objectives for triage are:
1. To perform a rapid primary and secondary survey of *all* patients who present to the ED for medical and nursing care.
2. To evaluate the patient's subjective complaint and the child's presenting signs and symptoms in order to assign the appropriate level of care classification.
3. To initiate appropriate emergency treatment measures, which include first aid, antipyretic therapy, and diagnostic studies according to the prescribed protocols.
4. To maintain a poised, controlled approach when communicating with families in need of crisis intervention.
5. To provide a caring and reassuring environment to children and their families during the initial phase of emergency care.

Pediatric Triage Assessment

Triage assessment of the pediatric patient is a rapid, focused 3 to 5 minute evaluation that includes the gathering of pertinent subjective and objective data to determine the child's severity of illness.

Triage evaluation includes subjective and objective assessment parameters such as the chief complaint, the child's level of consciousness, vital signs, mechanism of injury, obvious anatomic injury, and past medical history. In determining the child's severity of illness, *all* pertinent triage information must be gathered and analyzed as a collective whole to accurately assign the child an appropriate triage category: Critical, Acute, Urgent, or Nonurgent.

The Comprehensive Triage Process

The overall goal of triage is to rapidly assess the pediatric patient and determine the child's severity of illness. This initial screening and classification of the patient frequently determines how quickly the child will receive medical and nursing intervention. Because of the potential for rapid deterioration of the pediatric patient, a precise and accurate triage process is critical.

The comprehensive triage process is the most advanced system of triage and is supported by the Emergency Nurses Association Practice Standards. Assessment and prioritization of patients are performed by an educated, experienced RN (see Appendix A for triage nurse job description). The comprehensive triage process includes the evaluation and classification of all incoming patients to the ED, initiation of first aid measures, ordering diagnostic studies and procedures according to prescribed triage protocols, and performing ongoing patient reassessments.

The triage evaluation is completed by an experienced registered nurse who is stationed in the ED triage area 24 hours per day, 7 days per week for continuous coverage and availability to patients in need.

The ideal triage system ensures that all patients are seen immediately upon arrival to the ED. During periods of routine ED volumes, one triage nurse may be sufficient to evaluate incoming patients. However, during high volume periods it may be necessary to station a second "sorter" nurse in the triage area who also assists with patient assessment and screening.

The triage system that includes a primary nurse and a sorter nurse is considered a two-tiered triage system and is a novel approach to a comprehensive triage system during high volume periods. Some of the benefits to this system are:

1. Critical and acute patients can be identified more rapidly, thereby expediting emergency care.
2. ED triage waiting times are significantly decreased, which expedites patient flow into the emergency care system.
3. Patients who have or have been exposed to communicable diseases are identified sooner and placed on necessary isolation precautions.
4. Both triage nurses have a clear idea of patient acuity and chief complaints while waiting for further evaluation. (This information can then be communicated to the charge nurse and ED attending physician.)
5. Both the primary and sorter triage nurses can assist with patient reassessments, diagnostic studies, and triage procedures.

Primary and Secondary Triage Survey

The triage evaluation can be completed in an organized and systematic manner using the primary and secondary survey method endorsed by the American College of Surgeons Committee on Trauma.

The primary and secondary survey is a precise method to quickly and accurately assess a patient's severity of illness or injury. The Advanced Trauma Life Support (ATLS) method for completing the primary and secondary survey is widely used by prehospital and advanced trauma life support members nationwide. The concept of the primary and secondary survey has been modified and adapted for use by the triage nurse when evaluating all incoming patients to the hospital ED.

The primary survey consists of evaluating the child's airway, breathing, and circulation (A,B,Cs). The secondary survey is a more general head-to-toe assessment of the child's overall condition.

A simple method developed by the Emergency Nursing Pediatric Course uses a systematic approach for completing the primary and secondary survey and has been adapted in the box below. This method uses an A through J alphabetized mnemonic device to systematically assess the pediatric patient.

Primary and Secondary Pediatric Triage Survey

PRIMARY

A = Airway	✓ patency, positioning for air entry, audible sounds, airway obstruction (blood, mucous, edema, foreign body)
B = Breathing	✓ increased or decreased work of breathing, quality of breath sounds; nasal flaring; use of accessory muscles; pattern; quality; rate
C = Circulation	✓ color and temperature of skin; capillary refill, strength and rate of peripheral pulses
C = Cervical collar	placement of a cervical collar when indicated
C = Consciousness	✓ level of consciousness (Glasgow Coma Scale); response to environment; muscle tone; pupil response
D = Dextrose	✓ serum glucose level in patients with altered mental status
E = Expose	expose patient by undressing to identify underlying injuries

SECONDARY

F = Find	find out underlying history of current illness or injury
G = Get vital signs	obtain vital signs, obtain orthostatic vital signs if condition warrants
H = Head-to-toe assessment	perform a head-to-toe assessment for a complete and thorough examination
I = Initiate	initiate the Triage Documentation Record
I = Isolate	assess patient for rashes, communicable diseases, or immunosuppression, and place in appropriate isolation
I = Intervention	perform triage interventions (first aid, medication, administration, diagnostic studies)
J = Judgement	make appropriate triage classification of patient acuity

✓ = Check

Modified from *Pediatric emergency nursing resource guide*, Park Ridge, Ill, 1993, Emergency Nurses Association.

During the survey, the triage nurse immediately assesses A,B,C. If the child has cardiorespiratory instability, the triage assessment is *immediately* concluded and the child is brought directly to an emergency treatment area or resuscitation room where advanced life saving measures can be instituted.

The General Triage Interview

The triage interview is a three-way communication process between the nurse, child, and caretaker. This process is the basis for clinical judgments and decisions that are made regarding the child's severity of illness. Once the severity of illness is determined, appropriate medical and nursing interventions can be instituted.

The triage interview generally begins with the child's stated chief complaint. The triage nurse elicits pertinent subjective and objective information from the child and the caretaker to validate the child's severity of illness. The triage nurse must be skilled in asking specific developmentally appropriate questions in order to obtain the necessary history surrounding the current illness. See the following boxes for an outline of specific questions and a mnemonic device to elicit further information pertaining to the child's current illness or injury. Once the general interview and the primary and secondary survey are completed, the triage nurse concludes her evaluation and assigns the patient a triage category (Critical, Acute, Urgent, or Nonurgent). In addition, the triage nurse also documents pertinent findings on the Triage Record that include nursing assessments, vital signs, nursing interventions, significant historical information, diagnostic procedures, and medications administered (see Appendix C for triage record).

General Triage Interview

1. Patient name, age, and gender
2. Chief complaint (subjective)
3. Examination of current illness or injury
4. Mechanism of injury
5. Past medical history
6. Allergies
7. Current medications; time and amount of last dose
8. Immunization status
9. Exposure to communicable diseases
10. Mode of arrival

Modified from *Triage: meeting the challenge,* Park Ridge, Ill, 1992, Emergency Nurses Association.

P Q R S T Mnemonic

P (provokes)	What provokes the symptom?
Q (quality)	What makes it (the symptom) better or worse?
	What does it (the symptom) feel like?
R (radiation)	Where is it (the symptom)? Where does it radiate to?
S (severity)	If you could rate the symptom on a scale of 1 to 10 (1 = least, 10 = worst), how would you rate it?
T (time)	How long have you had this symptom? When did it start? When did it end? How long did it last?

Modified from Rice M, Abel C: Triage. In Buddasi, Sheehy: *Emergency nursing: practices and principles,* ed 3, St. Louis, 1992, Mosby.

The Psychosocial Triage Interview

Another important component of the triage process may include an assessment of the patient's psychosocial status. The confidential psychosocial triage interview includes the patient and the triage nurse. The interview may also include a caregiver, friend, relative, school liaison, religious advisor, or community health care provider. The triage nurse must be adept at asking specific questions surrounding a potentially life-threatening event in a confidential, caring manner. The box that follows describes various questions that can be used by the triage nurse to assist in the interview process.

The Suspected Child Abuse or Neglect (SCAN) Triage Interview

The assessment of a child for suspicious injuries and potential abuse is often quite difficult, requiring a multidisciplinary team approach. The triage nurse must be skilled as well as tactful in eliciting pertinent information surrounding the child's present and/or previous injury(s).

A consistent and thorough triage evaluation includes a primary and secondary survey, and a complete history of the event. Interview the child and the caretaker separately for comparison (refer to the following boxes for historical and physical indicators for abuse). Once data surrounding the event are collected, the triage nurse must carefully document, for medical and legal purposes, all essential information on the triage form; this information should include a description of the injury, size of the injury, color of the injury, mechanism of injury, person(s) present during the injury, time of the injury, and location of the injury. Carefully document behavioral and developmental actions exhibited by the child (eye contact, verbalization, exploration). Document specific quotes from the child and the caretaker pertaining to the event. In addition, document interactions between the caretaker and the child (e.g., Does the caretaker comfort the child? Does the child appear fearful of the caretaker?).

Psychosocial Triage Interview

1. What is the patient's perception or reason for the ED visit?
   - "What brings you to the emergency department today?"
2. Question the patient for presence of self-destructive thoughts:
   - "Have you ever thought about harming yourself?" **If yes, continue to question:**
   - "What would you want to happen if you did harm yourself?"
   - "Have you thought about how you might want to hurt yourself?"
   - "When did you last have these thoughts?" "How frequently?"
   - "Have you ever tried to hurt yourself in the past?" **If yes, describe.**
3. Question the patient for presence of disturbed thinking:
   - "Do you ever have thoughts that are disturbing or upsetting to you?" **If yes, describe.**
   - "Do you sometimes feel people are talking about you?"
   - "Do you ever hear people talking to you that you can't see?" **If yes, describe content.**
   - **If patient is preoccupied, gesturing, or posturing ask:** "Tell me what's happening right now?" or "What are you thinking?" "What's going through your head?"

Modified from Heller C, Knox-Fischer C: *Psychiatric emergency triage evaluation guidelines*, 1992, The Children's Hospital of Philadelphia.

Historical Indicators for Abuse

1. Is the history one of inflicted injury?
2. Is there an absence of history, a "magical injury?"
3. Could the injury have been avoided by better care and supervision?
4. Are there inconsistencies or changes in the history?
5. Is there a history of repeated injuries or hospitalizations?
6. Was there a delay in seeking medical care?
7. Does the history overestimate or underestimate the injury?
8. Is there a past medical history of prematurity, failure to thrive, failure to receive adequate medical care such as immunizations?

From Fleisher G, Ludwig S: *Textbook of pediatric emergency medicine,* Baltimore, 1993, Williams and Wilkins.

Physical Indicators for Abuse

1. Does the injury match the history?
2. Are there pathognomonic injuries such as looped wire marks or cigarette burns?
3. Are there multiple injuries?
4. Are there injuries at various stages of healing?
5. Are there different injury forms, for example, burns and fractures?
6. Is there evidence of overall poor care?
7. Has poisoning been documented in a young child?
8. Is there evidence of failure to thrive without a history of symptoms or physical findings?
9. Are there any visual or unexplained physical findings?

From Fleisher G, Ludwig S: *Textbook of pediatric emergency medicine,* Baltimore 1993, Williams and Wilkins.

Section II

Reference Data

▬ Normal Vital Signs and Parameters†

TABLE 1	**Normal Pediatric Vital Signs**				
	Vital signs				
	HEART RATE/ MIN, AWAKE	**HEART RATE/ MIN, ASLEEP**	**RESPIRATORY RATE/MIN**	**SYSTOLIC BP MMHG**	**DIASTOLIC BP MMHG**
Neonate	100–180	80–160	40–60	60–90	20–60
Infant (6 mo)	100–160	75–160	30–60	87–105	53–66
Toddler (2 yr)	80–110	60–90	24–40	95–105	53–66
Preschool (5 yr)	70–110	60–90	22–34	96–110	55–69
School age (7 yr)	65–110	60–90	18–30	97–112	57–71
Adolescent (15 yr)	60–90	50–90	12–16	112–128	66–80

BP, Blood pressure. Modified from *Textbook of pediatric advanced life support,* 1994, American Heart Association; Hazinski M. *Nursing care of the critically ill child,* St. Louis, 1992, Mosby; and Grossman M, Dieckmann R: *Pediatric emergency medicine,* Philadelphia, 1991, J.B. Lippincott.

Orthostatic Vital Signs

Orthostatic vital signs are defined as:
- A fall in systolic BP >25mmMg; a fall in diastolic BP >10 mmMg; signs and symtoms of inadequate cerebral prefusion; and compensated elevation in heart rate (HR) >20 beats/minute accompanied by a change from supine to vertical posture

From Memmer M: Acute orthostatic hypotension, *Heart Lung* 17 (2):134, 1988.

Normal Pediatric Parameters

- SpO_2 ≥ 95% in room air
- Capillary refill ≤2 sec in a normothermic patient
- Glasgow Coma Scale score ≥15 (see inside back cover for scoring)

†NOTE: These are normal values based on a patient without underlying pathology. It is normal for the heart rate and respiratory rate to increase in a patient with fever or stress.

■ Altered Respiratory Status

Severe Respiratory Distress

CRITICAL TRIAGE CATEGORY
- Cyanosis
- Agonal breath sounds
- Absent breath sounds
- Apnea >10 seconds
- Marked stridor (audible/loud)
- Marked wheezing
- Profound difficulty breathing
  - Marked retractions (supraclavicular, suprasternal, intercostal, subcostal)
  - Flaring
  - Grunting
  - Dyspnea
  - Shortness of breath (SOB)
  - Marked tachypnea

Moderate Respiratory Distress

ACUTE TRIAGE CATEGORY
- Persistent inspiratory/expiratory wheeze
- Noticeable stridor (audible/soft)
- Increased difficulty breathing
  - Moderate retractions
  - Flaring
  - Grunting
  - Dyspnea
  - SOB
- Significant tachypnea
- Decreased breath sounds

Mild Respiratory Distress

URGENT TRIAGE CATEGORY
- Intermittent inspiratory/expiratory wheeze
- Mild stridor (barely audible)
- Unequal breath sounds
- Mild tachypnea
- Mild retractions
- Rales

NOTE: The three categories for altered respiratory and hydration status are used in the various triage protocols in Section IV.

■ Altered Hydration Status

Severe Dehydration (>10%)

CRITICAL TRIAGE CATEGORY
- Unstable vital signs
  - Marked tachycardia
  - Marked hypotension
- Feeble or absent peripheral pulses
- Capillary refill >3 seconds (in normothermic patient)
- Cold, mottled extremities
- Stuporous, difficult to arouse
- Oliguria

Moderate Dehydration (5%–10%)

ACUTE TRIAGE CATEGORY
- Orthostatic vital signs (see p. 10)
  - Fall in systolic blood pressure (BP) >25 mmHg
  - Fall in diastolic BP >10 mmHg
  - Increased heart rate (HR) >20 beats/minute
  - Changes in sensorium
- Significant tachycardia
- Irritability, listlessness, lethargy
- Capillary refill 2–3 seconds
- Parched mucous membranes
- Sunken eyes/fontanel
- Tenting of skin
- Absent tears
- No urine output >12 hours

Mild Dehydration (3%–5%)

URGENT TRIAGE CATEGORY
- Mild tachycardia
- Cranky or restless
- Thirsty
- Slightly sunken eyes/fontanel
- Tacky mucous membranes
- Skin retracts slowly
- Reduced urine output
- Diminished tears

Modified from Fleisher G, Ludwig S: *Textbook of pediatric emergency medicine*, ed 3, Baltimore, 1993, Williams and Wilkins.

TABLE 2   Cranial Nerve Assessment and Function

Cranial Nerve Name	Function	Mechanism of Injury	Assessment Method
I. Olfactory	Smell	Fracture of cribiform plate or ethmoid area (rare)	Application of simple odors
II. Optic[†]	Vision	Direct trauma to orbit or globe; fracture involving optic foramen (relatively common); increased ICP	Ask child to describe objects near and far and also ask for identification of colors; test each eye separately and assess ability of child to see object moving into visual field from periphery
III. Oculomotor[†]	Pupil constriction, movement of eye and eyelid	Pressure of herniating uncus on nerve or fracture involving cavernous sinus	Both pupils should constrict in response to light as light is applied to each; consensual constriction (constriction in response to light directed to contralateral eye) should also be observed; eyes should be able to follow moving object throughout visual field, and eyelids should raise equally when eyes are open; ptosis and lateral downward deviation of eye with pupil dilation and decreased response to light are typical signs of oculomotor injury; always record pupil size in mm

Cranial Nerve Name	Function	Mechanism of Injury	Assessment
IV. Trochlear†	Movement of eye (superior oblique muscle)	Injury near course of nerve in area of brain stem or fracture of orbit (uncommon)	Assess ability of eyes to track object throughout visual field; damage to this nerve prevents eyes from moving downward and medically; diplopia may also be present
V. Trigeminal	Sensation to most of face and movement of jaw (mastication)	Direct injury to terminal branches, particularly to fibers of second division in roof of maxillary sinus	Apply soft and sharp objects to facial skin (with patient's eyes covered) and assess sensation (test above eye, upper lip, lower lip, and chin to test all three branches); motor functions are intact if child can clench and move jaw and chew food
VI. Abducens†	Lateral movement of eye	Injury near brain stem and course of nerve (uncommon)	Assess eye movement within socket by tracking an object throughout visual field; assess conjugate eye movement by moving object close to patient—both eyes should track object and move together as object is tracked throughout visual field
VII. Facial	Motor innervation (forehead, eyes, and mouth) and sensation to anterior two thirds of tongue (sweet/bitter discrimination); tearing	Fracture of temporal bone, laceration in area of parotid gland	Ask child to "make faces" and assess symmetry of face; test taste different on front of tongue; tearing with cry should be present

continued

TABLE 2	Cranial Nerve Assessment and Function–Continued		
Cranial Nerve Name	**Function**	**Mechanism of Injury**	**Assessment**
VIII. Vestibulocochlear (acoustic)	Hearing and equilibrium	Fracture of petrous portion of temporal bone (often injured in conjunction with cranial nerve VII)	Check gross hearing by clapping hands (startle and blink reflex should occur with sudden sound); test fine hearing using ticking watch or tuning fork; vestibular division is tested for "cold water calorics" and "doll's eyes" responses; both reflexes require that cranial nerve innervation controlling lateral gaze (cranial nerves III and VI) be intact for normal response; "cold water calorics" response involves instillation of cold water in ear to stimulate cranial nerves III, VI, and VIII, producing lateral nystagmus *(do not perform this test if patient is conscious*—this is typically performed to document absence of any cranial nerve function); "doll's eyes" maneuver also tests vestibular portion of cranial nerve VIII as well as cranial nerves III and VI (lateral gaze): as patient's head is turned, eyes should shift in sockets in direction *opposite* head rotation

Cranial Nerve Name	Function	Mechanism of Injury	Assessment
IX. Glossopharyngeal	Motor fibers to throat, voluntary muscles of swallowing, speech, taste to posterior one third of tongue	Brain stem injury or deep laceration of neck	Evaluate swallow, cough, and gag (tests cranial nerves IX and X simultaneously); clarity of speech should also be evaluated.
X. Vagus	Sensory and motor impulses for pharynx and parasympathetic fibers to abdomen	Brain stem injury, deep laceration of neck (rare)	Test as above, particularly cough and gag reflexes.
XI. Spinal accessory	Motor innervation of sternocleidomastoid, upper trapezius	Laceration of neck (rare)	Ask child to turn head as you palpate sternocleidomastoid and to shrug shoulders as you feel trapezius muscles contract.
XII. Hypoglossal	Innervation of tongue	Neck laceration associated with injury of major vessels	Ask child to stick out tongue; pinch nose of infant; mouth should open and tip of tongue should rise in midline

Modified from Hazinski M: *Nursing care of the critically ill child,* ed 2, St. Louis, 1992, Mosby.

†Innervation to eye muscles is generally tested simultaneously, and cranial nerves controlling lateral gaze (III and VI) *must* be intact to obtain a *normal* or *positive* "doll's eyes" response (oculocephalic reflex) and "cold water calorics" response (oculovestibular reflex).

Classification of Burn Injuries

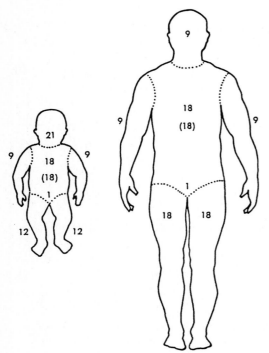

Lund and Browder Chart

Burned Area	1	1-4	5-9	10-14	15	Adult
			Total Body Surface			
Head	19 %	17 %	13 %	11 %	9 %	7 %
Neck	2	2	2	2	2	2
Anterior trunk	13	13	13	13	13	13
Posterior trunk	13	13	13	13	13	13
Right buttock	2.5	2.5	2.5	2.5	2.5	2.5
Left buttock	2.5	2.5	2.5	2.5	2.5	2.5
Genitalia	1	1	1	1	1	1
R.U. arm	4	4	4	4	4	4
L.U. arm	4	4	4	4	4	4
R.L. arm	3	3	3	3	3	3
L.L. arm	3	3	3	3	3	3
Right hand	2.5	2.5	2.5	2.5	2.5	2.5
Left hand	2.5	2.5	2.5	2.5	2.5	2.5
Right thigh	5.5	6.5	8	8.5	9	9.5
Left thigh	5.5	6.5	8	8.5	9	9.5
Right leg	5	5	5.5	6	6.5	7
Left leg	5	5	5.5	6	6.5	7
Right foot	3.5	3.5	3.5	3.5	3.5	3.5
Left foot	3.5	3.5	3.5	3.5	3.5	3.5

Figure 1

Lund and Browder chart: adult and child
(From Hazinski M: *Nursing care of the critically ill child*, 1992, St. Louis, Mosby.)

The Lund and Browder method is the most accurate and widely used formula for determining the extent of burn injury in adults and children. This method incorporates changes in the percentages of the child's total body surface area (TBSA) as the child grows.

TABLE 3   Common Skin Lesions

Primary lesions	Description	Example
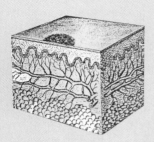 Macule	Flat circumscribed area of color change less than 1 cm in diameter, neither elevated nor depressed and with no alteration in skin texture	Freckle, nevus, measles
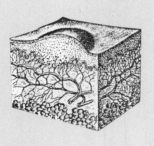 Papule	Small, circumscribed, solid elevation of the skin, less than 1 cm in diameter mostly above the plain of the skin surface, and the more superficial it is, the more distinct are the borders	Wart, ringworm
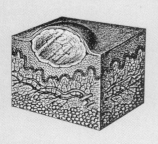 Nodule	Solid, circumscribed elevation, round or ellipsoid, located deep in dermis or subcutaneous tissue	Dermatofibroma

continued

TABLE 3	Common Skin Lesions—Continued	
Primary lesions	**Description**	**Example**
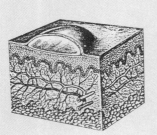\n\nVesicle	Small (less than 1 cm in diameter), superficial, circumscribed elevation of the skin containing serous or blood-tinged fluid	Chickenpox, herpes, poison ivy, dermatitis
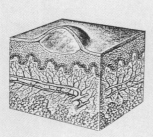\n\nPustule	Vesicle filled with pus that may not be caused by infection	Acne, impetigo, folliculitis
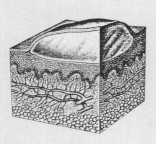\n\nBulla	Fluid-filled vesicle greater than 1 cm in diameter; a large vesicle; bleb; blister	Second-degree burn

Primary lesions	Description	Example
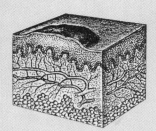 Wheal (hives)	Round or flat-topped and irregularly shaped, evanescent lesions resulting from acute accumulation of edema fluid in upper dermis	Mosquito bites, urticaria
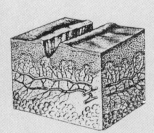 Excoriation or erosion	Superficial loss of skin substance that does not extend into dermis	Superficial scratches
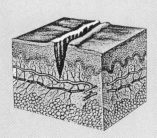 Fissure	Deep linear split through epidermis into dermis	Chapping

Modified from Thompson J et al: *Mosby's clinical nursing,* ed 3, St. Louis, 1993, Mosby.

TABLE 4 Common Skin Rashes

	Measles (rubeola)	Chickenpox (varicella)	Scarlet fever	Roseola (exanthem subitum)	Petechial rash from meningitis
Incubation	10–11 days	10–20 days	2–4 days	10–15 days	None
Signs and symptoms	3–5 days fever, cough, coryza, toxic appearance, conjunctivitis; Koplik's spots (mucosal lesions) appear 2 days before body rash	Fever and cough with rash; headache; malaise	Fever for 1–2 days, sore throat, strawberry tongue, vomiting, chills, malaise	Rapid rise of high fever lasting 3–4 days, in otherwise well child	May be sudden onset or preceded by fever and malaise; if sudden onset and accompanied by fever, may indicate sepsis
Exanthem (Rash)	Reddish brown; begins on face, spreads downward; confluent high on body, discrete lesions in lower portions; lasts 7–10 days	Vesicles appearing in crops on trunk, scalp, face, extremities; lesions in all stages of development	Punctate, sandpaper texture; blanches on pressure; appears first in flexor areas; rash lasts 7 days	Appears discrete, rose-colored; appears after fever; starting on chest and spreading to face	Reddish-purple vascular, *non-blanching* rash
Complications	Pneumonia, encephalitis, otitis media	Pneumonia, encephalitis, Reye's syndrome	Rheumatic heart disease	None	Sepsis, septic shock, long-term sequelae from increased intracranial pressure

	Measles (rubeola)	Chickenpox (varicella)	Scarlet fever	Roseola (exanthem subitum)	Petechial rash from meningitis
Management	Supportive; acetaminophen; isolate; prevention by vaccination	Supportive; acetaminophen, calamine lotion, diphenhydramine; isolate	Supportive; antibiotics; isolate	Supportive; acetaminophen, possibly antibiotics	Basic life support, advanced life support, immediate physician evaluation, liver function tests; isolate; if gradual onset and no fever, may be from blood dyscrasia or prolonged Valsalva's maneuver (cough, vomiting)

Modified from Sheehey S: *Emergency nursing principles and practice*, ed 3, St. Louis, 1992, Mosby.

Skeletal Anatomy

**Appendicular
Skeleton**

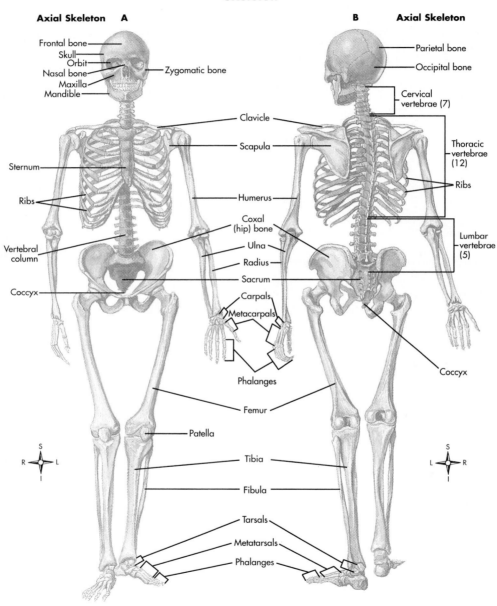

Axial Skeleton   **A**   **B**   **Axial Skeleton**

Frontal bone
Skull
Orbit
Nasal bone
Maxilla
Mandible
Zygomatic bone

Parietal bone
Occipital bone
Cervical
vertebrae (7)

Clavicle
Scapula
Thoracic
vertebrae
(12)

Sternum
Ribs

Ribs

Humerus

Vertebral
column

Coxal
(hip) bone
Ulna
Radius
Sacrum

Lumbar
vertebrae
(5)

Coccyx

Carpals
Metacarpals

Coccyx

Phalanges

Femur

Patella

Tibia

Fibula

Tarsals
Metatarsals
Phalanges

Figure 2

The complete skeleton. **A,** Anterior view. **B,** Posterior view.
(From Thibodeau GA, Patton KT: *Anthony's anatomy and physiology,* ed 15, St. Louis, 1996,
Mosby.)

Section III

Standing Triage Orders

Standing Medication Orders†

Acetaminophen

The triage nurse may administer acetaminophen (Tylenol) according to the following guidelines:

1. Patient's temperature is 38.3° C (101° F) or higher.
2. If acetaminophen was administered more than 2 hours earlier at home, another dose may be given in triage. This dose can be readministered within a short time.
3. Acetaminophen is contraindicated in patients with known hypersensitivity to acetaminophen or a history of liver disease.
4. For oral and rectal administration dose guidelines, see Table 5 or administer 10–15 mg/kg of acetaminophen based on the patient's **measured** weight.

	TABLE 5	Acetaminophen Dosing Guidelines	
Age	**Weight (lbs)**	**Weight (kg)**	**Dose (mg)**
0–3 mo	6–11	2.7–5	40
4–11 mo	12–17	5.4–7.7	80
12–23 mo	18–23	8.1–10.4	120
3 yr	24–35	10.9–15.9	160
4–5 yr	36–47	16.3–21.3	240
6–8 yr	48–59	21.8–26.8	320
9–10 yr	60–71	27.2–32.2	400
11 yr	72–95	32.7–43.2	480
12–14 yr	96 & over	43.6 & over	640

Modified from The Children's Hospital of Philadelphia, Penn, Emergency Department.

---

†The standing orders discussed in this section are suggested pediatric clinical practice protocols. In individual health care settings it may be necessary to develop or adapt these protocols to fit specific needs.

Ibuprofen

The triage nurse may administer ibuprofen according to the following guidelines:

1. Patients must receive an initial dose of acetaminophen at 10–15 mg/kg as the first line of antipyretic therapy before administering ibuprofen.
2. Patient's temperature is higher than 39.5° C (103.3° F) 1 hour after receiving an appropriate dose of acetaminophen according to the child's age and weight.
3. Patient is at least 6 months old.
4. Ibuprofen is contraindicated in patients with a medical history of chicken pox, asthma, ibuprofen or aspirin hypersensitivity, coagulopathy, emesis, moderate dehydration, or renal or liver disease. Ibuprofen is also contraindicated in patients less than 2 weeks postoperative because of prolonged bleeding times (e.g., after tonsil and adenoid surgery).
5. For oral administration dose guidelines, see Table 6 or administer 10 mg/kg of ibuprofen (children's Motrin or Advil) based on the patient's **measured** weight.

TABLE 6 **Ibuprofen Dosing Guidelines**

Age	Weight (lbs)	Weight (kg)	Dose (mg)
6–11 mo	13–16	5–7	50
12–23 mo	17–23	8–12	100
2–3 mo	24–35	13–17	150
4–5 yr	36–47	18–22	200
6–8 yr	48–59	23–27	250
9–10 yr	60–71	28–33	300
11–12 yr	72–95	32–44	400

Modified from The Children's Hospital of Philadelphia, Penn, Emergency Department.

Ibuprofen may be purchased over the counter and does not require a prescription.

Syrup of Ipecac

The triage nurse may administer syrup of ipecac under the following conditions:

1. Poison Control Center has been notified and recommends the administration of syrup of ipecac.
2. Patient is conscious and has a normal gag reflex.
3. Caretaker gives a reliable report that the ingestion occurred less than 30 minutes before triage evaluation.

The use of syrup of ipecac remains limited in the ED setting. It is generally **not** recommended for administration when emergency care can be promptly provided. Gastric lavage and charcoal administration are the preferred methods of gastric decontamination. However, syrup of ipecac can be administered in the prehospital setting when definitive care cannot be given in a timely manner (see Table 7).

LOCAL POISON CONTROL CENTER:

Phone: _____

TABLE 7	Syrup of Ipecac Dosing Guidelines		
Age	<12 mo	1–5 yr	≥5 yr
Dose	consult MD	15 ml	30 ml

Endorsed by The Poison Control Center, Philadelphia, Penn.

Standing Laboratory Orders

The triage nurse must use discretionary judgement in obtaining laboratory studies during high volume periods so as not to impede the care of other acutely ill children. The triage nurse may collect and send the following diagnostic laboratory studies when indicated:

Routine Urinalysis

A *clean catch* urinalysis may be collected from:
1. Any child or adolescent who reports signs or symptoms of urinary tract infections (UTIs).
2. Any child whose parent reports the child has had "UTI-like" signs or symptoms.
3. Any patient with abdominal pain, flank pain, or abdominal trauma.

Do not collect a urine specimen from any male with urethral discharge.

Urine Pregnancy

A *urine* pregnancy test may be collected from:
1. Any sexually active, postmenarchal female who complains of abdominal pain, spotting, or bleeding.
2. Any sexually active female who "suspects" that she may be pregnant, regardless of the chief complaint.
3. Any postmenarchal female before receiving any radiologic study.

Rapid Strep

A rapid strep test may be collected from:
1. Any patient with chief complaints of fever and sore throat.
2. Any patient with an exudative pharyngitis on oral examination.

▰ Standing Radiology Orders

The triage nurse may order diagnostic X-ray studies according to the following guidelines:

1. All potential fractures must be immobilized using a splint and/or sling before the X-ray study.
2. Any patient with an open fracture, a fracture causing neurovascular compromise, or multiple fractures should be triaged as "Critical"
3. *Do not* order X-ray studies if there is evidence of respiratory distress or if a more serious condition is suspected.
4. *Do not* delay necessary medical and nursing interventions when ordering diagnostic studies.
5. Consult the attending physician before ordering X-ray studies for any potentially pregnant female; send a urine pregnancy test for confirmation.
6. Consult the attending physician when uncertain of the specific X-ray study to order.

Foreign Body

X-ray studies may be ordered for:
1. Any patient with a laceration caused by glass.
2. Any patient who complains of *subcutaneous* glass or a metal foreign body that may be embedded in the tissue.
3. Consult the attending physician before ordering X-ray studies for any patient complaining of an ingested foreign body.

Orthopedic Injuries

The triage nurse may order X-ray studies of the following bones if there is:

1. Point tenderness or a clear deformity of the limb with significant swelling and decreased range of motion.

2. A history of trauma to the specific area less than 48 hours before arrival in the ED.

a) Clavicle	g) Hand
b) Shoulder	h) Finger
c) Humerus	i) Knee
d) Elbow	j) Tibia/fibula
e) Forearm	k) Ankle
f) Wrist	l) Foot

The following X-ray studies *should not* be ordered without first consulting the attending physician:

a) Spine	f) Chest
b) Scapula	g) Ribs
c) Skull	h) Abdomen
d) Facial bones	i) Hip
e) Soft tissue of the neck	j) Femur

During the triage examination if there is a marked diminished pulse distal to the injury, defer radiologic studies pending a consultation with the attending physician.

FRACTURES

For anatomic reference guide see Figure 2, *Skeletal Anatomy*, p. 22.

Section IV

Pediatric Triage Protocols

RESPIRATORY

Protocol 1 Apnea

Critical Triage	Acute Triage

Critical Triage

- **Any** critical vital sign/parameter (see inside back cover)
- Severe respiratory distress (see p. 11)

Acute Triage

- Moderate respiratory distress (see p. 11)
- Listless/lethargic
- History (Hx) of apnea *with* cyanotic episode at home
- Seizure ≤12 hours ago
- Seizure disorder
- Sibling of a child with Sudden Infant Death Syndrome (SIDS)

NOTE: This section consists of suggested pediatric clinical protocols. Individual health care settings may find it necessary to develop or adapt these protocols to fit their own specific needs.

Urgent Triage

- Mild respiratory distress (see p. 11)
- Reliable Hx of "stopped breathing" at home *without* cyanotic episode
- Increased apnea alarms on monitor *without* cyanotic event
- Hx of seizure >12 hours ago

Nonurgent Triage

- Stable cardiorespiratory status with:
  - * Breath-holding spell at home associated with crying
  - * Hx of coughing or gagging (turning red in face) *without* cyanotic episode

Interventions

- ◆ Complete primary (1°) and secondary (2°) survey (p. 3)
- ◆ ✓ Glasgow Coma Scale score (GCS) (see inside back cover)
- ◆ ✓ SpO$_2$ (pulse oximetry)
- ◆ ✓ for Hx of seizure or cyanosis surrounding the episode

RESPIRATORY

Protocol 2 Breathing Difficulty/Shortness of Breath

Critical Triage

- **Any** critical vital sign/parameter (see inside back cover)
- Severe respiratory distress (see p. 11)
- Unusual drooling, dysphagia, or dysphonia
- Unable to speak
- Marked hypertension
- Marked pallor
- Profusely diaphoretic
- Crushing chest pain radiating to jaw, neck, shoulder, back, or arms
- Irregular heartbeat
- Hx of being house fire victim or having faulty furnace in home

Acute Triage

- Moderate respiratory distress (see p. 11)
- Seizure ≤12 hours ago
- Listless/lethargic
- Muffled or distant heart tones
- Noticeable pallor
- Dizziness or syncopal episode
- Pleuritic chest pain
- Complaining of (c/o) heart beating fast, palpitations, or skipped beats
- Coughing up frank blood
- Hx of apneic episode at home
- Hx of chest trauma ≤12 hours ago
- Hx of choking episode at home on foreign body
- Hx of cyanotic episode at home
- Hx of ingestion of foreign substance
- SpO_2 93% to 94% in room air

Urgent Triage

- Mild respiratory distress (see p. 11)
- Chest discomfort that is *not* reproducible during sternal palpation or deep inhalation
- Rapid heartbeat with hyperventilation and c/o paresthesia
- Hx of chest trauma >12 hours ago

Nonurgent Triage

- Stable cardiorespiratory status with:
  - * Reproducible chest and sternal pain with sternal palpation and deep inhalation
  - * Rapid heartbeat with hyperventilation and *no* c/o paresthesia

Interventions

- ◆ Complete 1° and 2° survey (see p. 3)
- ◆ ✓ GCS (see inside back cover)
- ◆ ✓ SpO$_2$
- ◆ Auscultate heart rate (HR) for 60 seconds; note rate and rhythm
- ◆ Palpate sternum for reproducible chest pain associated with costochondritis

- ◆ Question caretaker for possible aspiration of foreign body or ingestion of foreign substance
- ◆ Give hyperventilating patient paper bag for rebreathing
- ◆ Consult physician (MD) for radiographic studies of neck, chest, or abdomen

RESPIRATORY

Protocol 3   Chest Trauma

Critical Triage

- **Any** critical vital sign/parameter (see inside back cover)
- Severe respiratory distress (see p. 11)
- Multiple traumatic injuries
- Marked pallor of mucous membranes
- Flail chest response
- Irregular heartbeat
- Crushing chest pain radiating to neck, jaw, shoulder, back, or arms
- Tracheal deviation

Acute Triage

- Moderate respiratory distress (see p. 11)
- Pleuritic chest pain
- Listless/lethargic
- Dizziness or syncopal episode
- Seizure ≤12 hours ago
- Hematemesis
- Hemoptysis
- Muffled or distant heart tones
- Weak peripheral pulses and cool extremities
- Possible rib or scapular fracture
- C/o fast heartbeat, palpitations, or skipped beats
- Subcutaneous emphysema of neck, chest, or clavicular area
- Cervical pain and tenderness with light palpation, or passive range of motion (ROM)

Urgent Triage

- Mild respiratory distress (see p. 11)
- Minor chest injury ≤12 hours ago
- Seizure >12 hours ago
- Clavicle fracture

Nonurgent Triage

- Stable cardiorespiratory status with minor chest injury >12 hours ago, and asymptomatic

Interventions

- Complete 1° and 2° survey (see p. 3)
- ✓ SpO₂
- ✓ GCS (see inside back cover)
- Auscultate HR for 60 seconds; note rate and rhythm
- Examine throat and neck for tracheal deviation

- Palpate neck, chest, and clavicle for subcutaneous air and crepitus
- Apply cervical collar on patients c/o cervical pain, and notify charge nurse or attending MD
- Complete trauma score (see Appendix C, p. 324)

RESPIRATORY

Protocol 4 Choking/Foreign Body Aspiration

Critical Triage

- **Any** critical vital sign/parameter (see inside back cover)
- Severe respiratory distress (see p. 11)
- Unusual drooling, dysphagia, or dysphonia
- Unable to speak

Acute Triage

- Moderate respiratory distress (see p. 11)
- Hx of cyanotic episode at home
- Persistent gagging, wretching, or coughing following a choking episode at home

Urgent Triage

- Mild respiratory distress (see p. 11)
- Reliable Hx of choking at home *without* cyanotic episode
- Localized pain in throat, chest, or abdomen

Nonurgent Triage

- Stable cardiorespiratory status with Hx of coughing or gagging at home (turning red) *without* drooling or cyanotic episode

Interventions

- ◆ Complete 1° and 2° survey (see p. 3)
- ◆ ✓ SpO$_2$
- ◆ Question caretaker about foreign body ingestion such as small coins or toys

RESPIRATORY

Protocol 5 Cough/Congestion

Critical Triage

- **Any** critical vital sign/parameter (see inside back cover)
- Severe respiratory distress (see p. 11)
- Unusual drooling, dysphagia, or dysphonia

Acute Triage

- Moderate respiratory distress (see p. 11)
- Paroxysmal cough followed by "whoop," or Hx of apneic episode at home
- Choking episode at home with persistent cough, gagging, or vomiting
- Coughing up frank blood
- Hx of apneic episode at home
- Hx of cyanotic episode at home
- Hx of cystic fibrosis

Urgent Triage

- Mild respiratory distress (see p. 11)
- Barking, "seal-like" cough
- Paroxysmal cough[†]

Nonurgent Triage

- Stable cardiorespiratory status with:
  * Mild cough
  * Rhinorrhea
  * Hx of gagging or coughing at home (turning red) *without* cyanotic episode

Interventions

- ◆ Complete 1° and 2° survey (see p. 3)
- ◆ ✓ for evidence of choking or possible aspiration of foreign body
- ◆ ✓ SpO$_2$
- ◆ ✓ quality of cough

[†]Isolate any patient with paroxysmal cough until pertussis is ruled out.

RESPIRATORY

Protocol 6 Hyperventilation

Critical Triage

- **Any** critical vital sign/parameter (see inside back cover)
- Severe respiratory distress (see p. 11)
- Stuporous, difficult to arouse

Acute Triage

- Moderate respiratory distress (see p. 11)
- Hx of syncopal episode
- Hx of toxic substance ingestion
- Extreme agitation or hysteria
- Severe chest pain
- Delirium/disorientation

Urgent Triage

- Mild respiratory distress (see p. 11)
- Moderate chest discomfort
- Hyperventilation *with* paresthesia
- Dizziness
- Abdominal pain
- Tremors
- Muscle pain or stiffness

Nonurgent Triage

- Stable cardiorespiratory status with:
  * Awake, alert, cooperative mental state
  * Hyperventilation *without* paresthesia

Interventions

- ◆ Complete 1° and 2° survey (see p. 3)
- ◆ ✓ GCS (see inside back cover)
- ◆ Treatment (Tx): Instruct patient to rebreath into a paper bag to increase CO_2 content in blood

RESPIRATORY

Protocol 7 Near Drowning

Critical Triage

- **Any** critical vital sign/parameter (see inside back cover)
- Severe respiratory distress (see p. 11)
- Stuporous, difficult to arouse

Acute Triage

- Mild to moderate respiratory distress (see p. 11)
- Listless/lethargic
- Hx of loss of consciousness
- Marked pallor
- SpO_2 93% to 94% in room air

Urgent Triage

- Awake, alert with productive cough and gag
- Irritable or agitated behavior

Nonurgent Triage

- Stable cardiorespiratory status

Interventions

- ◆ Complete 1° and 2° survey (see p. 3)
- ◆ ✓ GCS (see inside back cover)
- ◆ ✓ SpO_2

RESPIRATORY

Protocol 8   Rhinorrhea

Critical Triage	Acute Triage
• **Any** critical vital sign/parameter (see inside back cover)	• Moderate respiratory distress (see p. 11)
• Severe respiratory distress (see p. 11)	• Sx of moderate dehydration (see p. 11)
• Hx of nasal or facial trauma *with* clear or serosanguinous nasal drainage	• SpO_2 93% to 94% in room air
• Symptoms (Sx) of severe dehydration (see p. 11)	• Fever ≥41° C oral or rectal
	• Fever ≥38° C rectal in infants ≤10 weeks old

Urgent Triage

- Mild respiratory distress (see p. 11)
- Sx of mild dehydration (see p. 11)
- Foul smelling, purulent rhinorrhea *with* facial tenderness
- Fever ≥38° C to 40.9° C rectal in infants 10 to 12 weeks old

Nonurgent Triage

- Stable cardiorespiratory and hydration status with:
  * Upper respiratory tract infection
  * Cough
  * Thin, watery discharge from nose
  * Fever ≥38° C to 40.9° C oral or rectal in infants >12 weeks old

Interventions

- ◆ Complete 1° and 2° survey (see p. 3)
- ◆ ✓ SpO_2
- ◆ Administer antipyretics for fever according to standing orders (see pp. 24 and 25)

RESPIRATORY

Protocol 9 Stridor

Critical Triage

- **Any** critical vital sign/parameter (see inside back cover)
- Unusual drooling, dysphagia, or dysphonia
- Severe respiratory distress (see p. 11)
- Sx of severe dehydration (see p. 11)

Acute Triage

- Moderate respiratory distress (see p. 11)
- Sx of moderate dehydration (see p. 11)
- Fever ≥41° C rectal or oral
- Fever ≥38° C rectal in infants ≤10 weeks old
- Foreign body in mouth, pharynx, or esophagus
- Hx of throat trauma ≤12 hours ago
- Muffled voice
- Listless/lethargic
- SpO_2 93% to 94% in room air

Urgent Triage

- Mild respiratory distress (see p. 11)
- Sx of mild dehydration (see p. 11)
- Fever ≥38° C to 40.9° C rectal in infants 10 to 12 weeks old
- Hx of throat trauma >12 hours ago
- Grossly enlarged tonsils

Nonurgent Triage

- Stable cardiorespiratory and hydration status with:
  * Minor upper respiratory tract infection *with* cough
  * Fever ≥38° C to 40.9° C rectal or oral in children >12 weeks old

Interventions

- ◆ Complete 1° and 2° survey (see p. 3)
- ◆ ✓ SpO$_2$
- ◆ Keep patient seated upright in a comfortable position
- ◆ Administer antipyretics for fever according to standing orders (see pp. 24 and 25)

RESPIRATORY

Protocol 10 Wheezing

Critical Triage	**Acute Triage**

Critical Triage

- **Any** critical vital sign/parameter (see inside back cover)
- Severe respiratory distress (see p. 11)
- Stuporous, difficult to arouse
- Sx of severe dehydration (see p. 11)
- Hx of being house fire victim or having faulty furnace in home
- Swelling of face, tongue, or lips

Acute Triage

- Moderate respiratory distress (see p. 11)
- Hx of foreign body aspiration
- Sx of moderate dehydration (see p. 11)
- Listless/lethargic
- Extreme irritability or agitation
- Chest pain
- Fever ≥41° C oral or rectal
- Fever ≥38° C rectal in infants ≤10 weeks old
- SpO_2 93% to 94% in room air

Urgent Triage

- Mild respiratory distress (see p. 11)
- Fever ≥38° C to 40.9° C rectal in infants 10 to 12 weeks old
- Sx of mild dehydration (see p. 11)

Nonurgent Triage

- Stable cardiorespiratory and hydration status with:
  - * Upper respiratory tract infection
  - * Rhinorrhea
  - * Fever ≥38° C to 40.9° C oral or rectal in children >12 weeks old
  - * Nasal congestion

Interventions

- ◆ Complete 1° and 2° survey (see p. 3)
- ◆ ✓ SpO_2
- ◆ Administer antipyretics for fever according to standing orders (see pp. 24 and 25)
- ◆ ✓ Hx for allergic reaction to foods or medications

CARDIOVASCULAR

Protocol **11**   Cardiac Dysfunction with Known Heart Disease

Critical Triage

- **Any** critical vital sign/parameter (see inside back cover)
- Cyanosis (new onset)
- Severe respiratory distress (see p. 11)
- Marked hypertension
- Irregular heartbeat
- Profusely diaphoretic
- Crushing chest pain radiating to jaw, neck, shoulder, back, or arms

Acute Triage

- Moderate respiratory distress (see p. 11)
- Listless/lethargic
- Muffled or distant heart tones
- Weak peripheral pulse and cool extremities
- +JVD (jugular venous distention) in older children when sitting upright
- Generalized edema
- Pleuritic chest pain
- C/o fast heart beat, palpitations, or skipped beats
- Dizziness or syncopal episode
- Increased cyanosis with congenital heart disease
- Fever ≥41° C oral or rectal

Urgent Triage

- Mild respiratory distress (see p. 11)
- Fever 38.3° C to 40.9° C oral or rectal
- Failure to thrive, poor feeding, poor weight gain

Nonurgent Triage

- Stable cardiorespiratory status with:
  * Cold or cough symptoms
  * Fever <38.3° C oral or rectal

Interventions

- ◆ Complete 1° and 2° survey (see p. 3)
- ◆ ✓ SpO_2
- ◆ Palpate sternum for reproducible chest pain
- ◆ Auscultate HR for 60 seconds; note rate and rhythm
- ◆ Administer antipyretics for fever according to standing orders (see pp. 24 and 25)

CARDIOVASCULAR

Protocol 12 Cardiac Dysfunction Without Hx of Heart Disea

Critical Triage

- **Any** critical vital sign/parameter (see inside back cover)
- Severe respiratory distress (see p. 11)
- Marked hypertension
- Irregular heartbeat
- Marked pallor
- Profusely diaphoretic
- Crushing chest pain radiating to jaw, neck, shoulder, back, or arms

Acute Triage

- Moderate respiratory distress (see p. 11)
- Listless/lethargic
- Muffled or distant heart tones
- Cool extremities, weak peripheral pulse
- Noticeable pallor
- +JVD in older children when sitting upright
- Hx chest trauma ≤12 hours ago
- Generalized edema
- Dizziness or syncopal episode
- Pleuritic chest pain
- C/o fast heartbeat, palpitations, or skipped beats

Urgent Triage

- Mild respiratory distress (see p. 11)
- Chest discomfort *not* reproducible during sternal palpation or deep inhalation
- Rapid HR with hyperventilation and c/o paresthesia
- Hx chest trauma 12 to 24 hours ago

Nonurgent Triage

- Stable cardiorespiratory status with:
  * Chest trauma ≥24 hours ago; asymptomatic
  * Reproducible sternal pain with sternal palpation and/or deep inhalation
  * Rapid heartbeat with hyperventilation and *no* c/o paresthesia

Interventions

- ◆ Complete 1° and 2° survey (p. 3)
- ◆ Palpate sternum for reproducible chest pain associated with costochondritis
- ◆ Auscultate HR for 60 seconds; note rate and rhythm
- ◆ ✓ SpO_2
- ◆ Give hyperventilating patients paper bag for rebreathing

CARDIOVASCULAR

Protocol 13 Chest Pain

Critical Triage

- **Any** critical vital sign/parameter (see inside back cover)
- Severe respiratory distress (see p. 11)
- Marked hypertension
- Irregular heartbeat
- Marked pallor
- Profusely diaphoretic
- Crushing chest pain radiating to jaw, neck, shoulder, back, or arms

Acute Triage

- Moderate respiratory distress (see p. 11)
- Listless/lethargic
- Muffled or distant heart tones
- Cool extremities, weak peripheral pulse
- Noticeable pallor
- +JVD in older children when sitting upright
- Generalized edema
- Dizziness or syncopal episode
- Hx of chest trauma ≤12 hours ago
- Pleuritic chest pain
- C/o fast heartbeat, palpitations, or skipped beats
- Hx of cystic fibrosis
- Hx of asthma
- Hx of sickle cell disease
- Hx of known cardiac disease
- Hx of Kawasaki syndrome
- Hx of Marfan's syndrome

Urgent Triage

- Mild respiratory distress (see p. 11)
- Chest discomfort that is *not* reproducible during sternal palpation or deep inhalation
- Rapid heartbeat with hyperventilation and c/o paresthesia
- Hx chest trauma 12 to 24 hours ago
- Fever ≥38.3° C oral or rectal
- Chest pain with exertion or exercise

Nonurgent Triage

- Stable cardiorespiratory status with:
  * Chest trauma >24 hours ago; asymptomatic at time of exam
  * Reproducible chest and sternal pain with sternal palpation and/or deep inhalation
  * Rapid heartbeat with hyperventilation and no c/o paresthesia

Interventions

- Complete 1° and 2° survey (see p. 3)
- Palpate sternum for reproducible chest pain associated with costochondritis
- Auscultate HR for 60 seconds; note rate and rhythm

- ✓ SpO_2
- Give hyperventilating patients paper bag for rebreathing

CARDIOVASCULAR

Protocol 14 Hypertension

Critical Triage

- **Any** critical vital sign/parameter (see inside back cover)
- Severe respiratory distress (see p. 11)
- Marked hypertension:
  - * SBP ≥160 if ≤10 yrs old
    SBP ≥170 if >10 yrs old

  - * DBP ≥105 if ≤10 yrs old
    DBP ≥110 if >10 yrs old
- Facial drooping, motor weakness, or slurred speech
- Profusely diaphoretic
- Crushing chest pain radiating to jaw, neck, shoulder, arms, or back
- Irregular heartbeat

Acute Triage

- Significant hypertension:
  - * DBP ≥86 if ≤9 yrs old
  - * DPB ≥90 if 10–15 yrs old
  - * DPB ≥98 if >15 yrs old
- Moderate respiratory distress (see p. 11)
- Agonizing headache
- Dizziness or syncopal episode
- Listless/lethargic
- Pleuritic chest pain
- C/o fast heartbeat, palpitations, or skipped beats
- Generalized edema
- Visual disturbances
- Seizure ≤12 hours ago
- Severe active bleeding from nose or mouth
- Hx of significant head trauma ≤12 hours ago
- Hx of toxic substance ingestion
- Hx of malignant hypertension
- Hx of renal disease or adrenal disease

DBP, Diastolic blood pressure; *SBP*, Systolic blood pressure.

Urgent Triage

- Mild respiratory distress (see p. 11)
- Seizure >12 hours ago
- Persistent headache
- Hx of minor head trauma ≤12 hours ago
- Intermittent epistaxis
- Nausea or vomiting

Nonurgent Triage

- Stable cardiorespiratory and neurologic status with:
  * Stable vital signs, including blood pressure (BP) (see p. 10)
  * Alert, awake, cooperative mental state

Interventions

- ◆ Complete 1° and 2° survey (see p. 3)
- ◆ Active nosebleed:
  * Tilt head forward; apply direct external pressure to nose for 5 to 10 min; and insert a cotton (dental) roll under upper lip to compress labial artery

- ◆ ✓ GCS (see inside back cover)
- ◆ Auscultate HR for 60 seconds; note rate and rhythm
- ◆ Use appropriate size BP cuff: Bladder size should equal 75% of upper length of arm to elbow

CARDIOVASCULAR

Protocol 15   Hypotension

Critical Triage

- **Any** critical vital sign/parameter (see inside back cover)
- Sx of severe dehydration (see p. 11)
- Petechial/purpuric rash *below* nipple line with fever ≥38.3° C oral or rectal*

Acute Triage

- Orthostatic vital signs (see p. 10)
- Sx of moderate dehydration (see p. 11)
- Fever ≥41° C oral or rectal
- Petechial or purpuric rash *below* nipple line with fever ≤38.3° C oral or rectal*
- Dizziness or syncopal episode
- Dextrose stick 40 to 80 mg/dl
- Teenage pregnancy
- Listless/lethargic

Urgent Triage

- Sx of mild dehydration (see p. 11)
- Hx of fainting before arrival in emergency department (ED)
- Petechial or purpuric rash *above* nipple line; afebrile[†]

Nonurgent Triage

- Stable cardiorespiratory, hydration, and neurologic status with:
  * Decreased oral fluid intake
  * Awake, alert, cooperative mental status

Interventions

- ◆ Complete 1° and 2° survey (see p. 3)
- ◆ ✓ GCS (see inside back cover)
- ◆ ✓ glucose via finger stick
- ◆ Administer ammonia smelling salts for syncopal episode

[†]Place in respiratory isolation

CARDIOVASCULAR

Protocol 16   Pacemaker Dysfunction

Critical Triage

- **Any** critical vital sign/parameter (see inside back cover)
- Severe respiratory distress (see p. 11)
- Marked hypertension
- Irregular heartbeat
- Marked pallor
- Profusely diaphoretic
- Crushing chest pain radiating to jaw, neck, shoulder, back, or arms

Acute Triage

- Moderate respiratory distress (see p. 11)
- Listless/lethargic
- Muffled or distant heart tones
- Cool extremities, weak peripheral pulses
- Noticeable pallor
- +JVD in older children when sitting upright
- Generalized edema
- Dizziness or syncopal episode
- Pleuritic chest pain
- C/o fast heartbeat, palpitations, or skipped beats

Urgent Triage

- Mild respiratory distress (see p. 11)
- Fever ≥38.3° C oral or rectal
- Chest discomfort *not* reproducible during sternal palpation or deep inhalation

Nonurgent Triage

- Stable cardiorespiratory status
- Triage other Sx

Interventions

- ◆ Complete 1° and 2° survey (see p. 3)
- ◆ ✓ GCS (see inside back cover)
- ◆ Auscultate HR for 60 seconds; note rate and rhythm; place on cardiac monitor as soon as possible

- ◆ Palpate sternum for reproducible chest pain associated with costo-chondritis
- ◆ ✓ SpO$_2$

NEUROLOGIC

Protocol 17 Altered Mental Status

Critical Triage

- **Any** critical vital sign/parameter (see inside back cover)
- Stuporous, difficult to arouse
- Slurred speech
- Generalized motor or sensory weakness
- Facial drooping or asymmetry
- Debilitating headache
- Marked hypertension

Acute Triage

- Confused, unable to follow commands
- Photophobia
- Severe headache
- Stiff neck/nuchal rigidity[†]
- Bulging anterior fontanel
- Visual impairment
- Persistent vomiting
- Focal motor or sensory weakness
- Seizure <12 hours ago
- Dextrose stick 40 to 80 mg/dl
- Displaying hostile or aggressive behavior[†]
- Hx of head trauma ≤12 hours ago
- Hx of toxic substance ingestion ≤24 hours ago
- Hx of ventroperitoneal (VP) shunt

Urgent Triage

- Painful headache
- Syncopal episode before arrival
- Sudden behavioral changes
- Seizure >12 hours ago
- Agitated behavior or suicidal ideation[††]
- Medical clearance for psychiatric admission
- Hx of psychiatric disorder
- Hx of minor head trauma >12 hours ago
- Hx of ingestion >24 hours ago

Nonurgent Triage

- Stable cardiorespiratory and neurologic status with awake, alert, cooperative mental status

Interventions

- ◆ Complete 1° and 2° survey (see p. 3)
- ◆ ✓ GCS (see inside back cover)
- ◆ ✓ pupils
- ◆ ✓ hand grasps and symmetry of smile
- ◆ ✓ glucose via finger stick

[†]Place in respiratory isolation.

[††]Aggressive suicidal patients need placement in private room with one-to-one supervision

NEUROLOGIC

Protocol **18** Ataxia

Critical Triage

- **Any** critical vital sign/parameter (see inside back cover)
- Stuporous, difficult to arouse
- Slurred speech
- Generalized motor or sensory weakness
- Facial drooping or asymmetry
- Debilitating headache

Acute Triage

- Confused, unable to follow commands
- Photophobia
- Severe headache
- Stiff neck/nuchal rigidity[†]
- Bulging anterior fontanel
- Staggering gait
- Visual impairment
- Persistent vomiting
- Focal motor or sensory weakness
- Seizure <12 hours ago
- Acute hearing loss
- Hx of brain tumor
- Hx of head trauma
- Hx of toxic substance ingestion
- Hx of ventroperitoneal shunt
- Dextrose stick 40 to 80 mg/dl

Urgent Triage	Nonurgent Triage
• Painful headache • Vertigo • Intermittent vomiting • Hyperventilation *with* paresthesia • Progressive hearing loss • Syncopal episode before arrival in ED • Seizure >12 hours ago • Sudden behavioral changes	• Stable cardiorespiratory and neurologic status with: * Awake, alert, cooperative mental status * Steady gait * Hyperventilation *without* paresthesia

Interventions

◆ complete 1° and 2° survey (see p. 3)

◆ ✓ GCS (see inside back cover)

◆ ✓ pupils

◆ ✓ gait

◆ ✓ gross motor and sensory functions

◆ ✓ glucose via finger stick

◆ ✓ hand grips and symmetry of smile

†Place in respiratory isolation.

NEUROLOGIC

Protocol 19 Crying/Irritability

Critical Triage

- **Any** critical vital sign/parameter (see inside back cover)
- Severe respiratory distress (see p. 11)
- Sx of severe dehydration (see p. 11)
- Stuporous, difficult to arouse
- Petechial or purpuric rash *below* nipple line with fever ≥38.3° C†
- Unrelenting irritability

Acute Triage

- Moderate respiratory distress (see p. 11)
- Sx of moderate dehydration (see p. 11)
- Petechial/purpuric rash below nipple line *with* fever <38.3° C†
- Fever ≥38° C rectal in infants ≤10 weeks old
- Fever ≥41° C oral or rectal
- Stiff neck/nuchal rigidity†
- Bulging anterior fontanel
- Severe headache
- High-pitched cry
- Inconsolable irritability
- Listless/lethargic
- Positive blood culture from previous visit
- Bilious vomiting

Urgent Triage

- Mild respiratory distress (see p. 11)
- Sx of mild dehydration (see p. 11)
- Fever ≥38° C to 40.9° C rectal in infants 10 to 12 weeks old
- Neonate with noticeable irritability and change in sleeping pattern

Nonurgent Triage

- Stable cardiorespiratory and neurologic status with:
  * Crying but consolable
  * Hx of colic
  * Teething
  * Fever ≥38° C to 40.9° C oral or rectal in children >12 weeks old

Interventions

- ◆ Complete 1° and 2° survey (see p. 3)
- ◆ ✓ GCS (see inside back cover)
- ◆ ✓ for petechial or purpuric rash
- ◆ Administer antipyretics for fever according to standing orders (see pp. 24 and 25)

---

†Place in respiratory isolation

NEUROLOGIC

Protocol **20** Fainting

Critical Triage	Acute Triage

Critical Triage

- **Any** critical vital sign/parameter (see inside back cover)
- Severe respiratory distress (see p. 11)
- Stuporous, difficult to arouse
- Sx of severe dehydration (see p. 11)

Acute Triage

- Orthostatic vital signs (see box on p. 10)
- Moderate respiratory distress (see p. 11)
- Sx of moderate dehydration (see p. 11)
- Hx of toxic substance ingestion <24 hours ago
- Listless/lethargic
- Confused, unable to follow commands
- Dextrose stick 40 to 80 mg/dl
- Marked pallor
- Extreme hysteria or emotional instability
- Hx of cardiac disease
- Hx of metabolic disease

Urgent Triage

- Moderate respiratory distress (see p. 11)
- Sx of moderate dehydration (see p. 11)
- Hyperventilation
- Hx of breath holding episode
- Hx of psychiatric disorder

Nonurgent Triage

- Stable cardiorespiratory and neurologic status with awake, alert, cooperative mental status

Interventions

- ◆ Complete 1° and 2° survey (see p. 3)
- ◆ ✓ GCS (see inside back cover)
- ◆ ✓ pupils
- ◆ ✓ glucose via finger stick

- ◆ Give hyperventilating patient paper bag for rebreathing

NEUROLOGIC

Protocol 21   Headache

Critical Triage

- **Any** critical vital sign/parameter (see inside back cover)
- Debilitating headache
- Stuporous, difficult to arouse
- Slurred speech
- Facial drooping or asymmetry
- Marked hypertension:
    * SBP ≥160 if ≤10 years old
      SBP ≥170 if >10 years old
    * DBP ≥105 if ≤10 years old
      DBP ≥110 if >10 years old

Acute Triage

- Significant hypertension:
    * DBP ≥86 if ≤9 years old
    * DBP ≥90 if 10–15 years old
    * DBP ≥98 if >15 years old
- Inconsolable irritability
- Listless/lethargic
- Confused, unable to follow commands
- Severe headache
- Persistent vomiting
- Stiff neck/nuchal rigidity[†]
- Visual impairment
- Seizure ≤12 hours ago
- Focal motor or sensory weakness
- Hx of brain tumor
- Hx of significant head trauma ≤12 hours ago
- Hx of ventroperitoneal shunt

Urgent Triage

- Sx of moderate dehydration (see p. 11)
- Seizure >12 hours ago
- Painful headache
- Hx of minor head trauma <12 hours ago
- Noticeable irritability

Nonurgent Triage

- Stable cardiorespiratory and neurologic status with:
  * Awake, alert, cooperative mental status
  * Mild headache
  * Hx of minor head injury >12 hours ago *without* vomiting

Interventions

- ◆ Complete 1° and 2° survey (see p. 3)
- ◆ ✓ GCS (see inside back cover)
- ◆ ✓ pupils
- ◆ Assess vital signs for increased intracranial pressure (ICP) and Cushing's triad:
  * ↑ SBP
  * Bradycardia
  * Widening pulse pressure

---

†Place in respiratory isolation.

NEUROLOGIC

Protocol 22   Head Trauma

Critical Triage

- **Any** critical vital sign/parameter (see inside back cover)
- Stuporous, difficult to arouse
- Severe respiratory distress (see p. 11)
- Hx of severe inherited bleeding disorder (e.g., hemophiliac)
- Large scalp laceration with pulsatile bleeding
- Multiple traumatic injuries
- Unequal or nonreactive pupils
- Facial drooping, motor or sensory weakness, slurred speech
- Cervical pain and tenderness with palpation or passive ROM
- Active clear fluid leak from ear or nose

Acute Triage

- Moderate respiratory distress (see p. 11)
- Head trauma with loss of consciousness or persistent vomiting
- Amnesia, inconsolable irritability
- Listless/lethargic
- Multiple unexplained bruises, contusions, or lacerations
- Seizure ≤12 hours ago
- Battle's sign (eccyhmosis behind ear)
- Raccoon eyes (periorbital ecchymosis)
- Depressed skull fracture (Fx) with palpation of step-off
- Agonizing headache
- Visual impairment
- Dizziness or syncopal episode
- Large scalp or facial laceration ≤12 hours ago

Urgent Triage

- Mild respiratory distress (see p. 11)
- Minor head trauma ≤12 hours ago *without* loss of consciousness or vomiting
- Localized unexplained bruises, contusions, or lacerations
- Seizure >12 hours ago
- Hematuria
- Scalp or facial laceration ≤12 hours ago
- Intense headache
- Sudden behavioral changes
- Noticeable irritability

Nonurgent Triage

- Stable cardiorespiratory and neurologic status with:
  * Minor head injury >12 hours ago *without* loss of consciousness or vomiting
  * Minor scalp or facial laceration >12 hours ago
  * Awake, alert, cooperative mental status

Interventions

- Complete 1° and 2° survey (see p. 3)
- ✓ GCS (see inside back cover)
- Apply cervical collar to patients c/o cervical pain and notify charge nurse or attending MD
- Apply normal sterile saline (NSS) pressure dressing to open wounds
- ✓ pupils and extraocular muscle function

- Apply ice to hematoma
- Keep NPO if vomiting
- Keep NPO if ≥ Urgent triage category
- Assess vital signs for ↑ICP and Cushing's triad:
  * ↑SBP
  * Bradycardia
  * Widening pulse pressure
- Complete trauma score (see Appendix C)

NEUROLOGIC

Protocol 23   Seizure

Critical Triage	**Acute Triage**
• **Any** critical vital sign/parameter (see inside back cover)	• Moderate respiratory distress (see p. 11)
• Severe respiratory distress (see p. 11)	• Sx of moderate dehydration (see p. 11)
• Stuporous, difficult to arouse	• Temperature ≥38.3° C oral or rectal
• Sx of severe dehydration (see p. 11)	• Stiff neck/nuchal rigidity†
	• Seizure ≤12 hours ago
	• Dextrose stick 40 to 80 mg/dl
	• Inconsolable irritability
	• Listless/lethargic
	• Hx of toxic substance ingestion
	• Hx of head trauma
	• Hx of ventroperitoneal shunt
	• Hx of seizure disorder

Urgent Triage

- Mild respiratory distress (see p. 11)
- Sx of mild dehydration (see p. 11)
- Hx of seizure >12 hours ago

Nonurgent Triage

- Stable cardiorespiratory and neurologic status
- Triage other Sx

Interventions

- ◆ Complete 1° and 2° survey (see p. 3)
- ◆ ✓ GCS (see inside back cover)
- ◆ ✓ SpO$_2$
- ◆ ✓ glucose via finger stick
- ◆ Administer antipyretics for fever according to standing orders (see pp. 24 and 25)

---

†Place in respiratory isolation.

NEUROLOGIC

Protocol 24 Ventriculoperitoneal (VP) Shunt Malfunction

Critical Triage

- **Any** critical vital sign/parameter (see inside back cover)
- Stuporous, difficulty to arouse
- Generalized motor and sensory weakness
- Debilitating headache

Acute Triage

- Fever ≥38.3° C oral or rectal
- Marked irritability
- Listless/lethargic
- Intense headache
- Stiff neck/nuchal rigidity[†]
- Bulging anterior fontanel
- Visual impairment
- Photophobia
- Persistent vomiting
- Abdominal pain and tenderness
- Seizure ≤12 hours ago
- Hx of brain tumor
- Hx of hydrocephalus

Urgent Triage

- Mild headache
- Intermittent vomiting
- Seizure >12 hours ago
- Sleepy but easily arousable
- New onset of redness or swelling around shunt site or bubble *without* fever

Nonurgent Triage

- Stable cardiorespiratory, hydration, and neurologic status with awake, alert, cooperative mental status

Interventions

- ◆ Complete 1° and 2° survey (see p. 3)
- ◆ ✓ GCS (see inside back cover)
- ◆ ✓ pupils
- ◆ Assess vital signs for ↑ICP and Cushing's triad:
    - * ↑SBP
    - * Bradycardia
    - * Widening pulse pressure

†Place in respiratory isolation

EYE

Protocol 25 Eye Foreign Substance

Critical Triage

- **Any** critical vital sign/parameter (see inside back cover)
- Penetrating injury to eye
- Chemical substance or smoke burn to eye
- Eye laceration with or without hyphema
- Ruptured globe

Acute Triage

- Hyphema
- Visual impairment
- Obvious foreign body in eye
- Dizziness or syncopal episode
- Cloudy vision with flashing lights or curtain in visual field
- Pupil abnormalities

Urgent Triage

- Moderate eye irritation with pain
- Unable to open eye spontaneously
- Considerable swelling or tearing of eye

Nonurgent Triage

- Stable cardiorespiratory and neurologic status with:
  * Visual acuity and extraocular muscles intact
  * Minor eye irritation with redness or tearing

Interventions

- ◆ Complete 1° and 2° survey (p. 3)
- ◆ ✓ pupils
- ◆ ✓ visual acuity
- ◆ ✓ extraocular movement
- ◆ Place eye shield or soft patch over affected eye

- ◆ Ask patient if he/she wears contact lenses
- ◆ Ask patient if foreign body was metallic substance

EYE

Protocol 26 Eye Redness/Drainage

Critical Triage

- **Any** critical vital sign/parameter (see inside back cover)
- Severe respiratory distress (see p. 11)
- Penetrating injury to eye
- Chemical substance or smoke burn to eye

Acute Triage

- Moderate respiratory distress (see p. 11)
- Foreign body in eye
- Significant trauma to eye ≤12 hours ago
- Hyphema
- Visual impairment
- Periorbital swelling and redness *with* fever ≥38° C rectal in infants ≤10 weeks old
- Fever ≥41° C rectal or oral

Urgent Triage

- Mild respiratory distress (see p. 11)
- Periorbital swelling and redness with fever <38° C to 40.9° C rectal in infants 10 to 12 weeks old
- Minor trauma to eye ≤12 hours ago
- Moderate eye irritation with pain
- Photophobia
- Copious purulent eye discharge with tenderness

Nonurgent Triage

- Stable cardiorespiratory status with:
  * Visual acuity and extraocular muscles intact
  * Conjunctivitis/iritis/uveitis
  * Minor clear to yellow eye discharge
    –Eye tearing
    –Eye itching
- Fever 38° C to 40.9° C oral or rectal in infants >12 weeks old

Interventions

- Complete 1° and 2° survey (p. 3)
- Assess visual acuity
- Place eye shield or soft patch over affected eye

- Ask patient if he/she wears contact lenses
- Administer antipyretics for fever according to standing orders (see pp. 24 and 25)

EYE

Protocol 27 Eye Swelling

Critical Triage

- **Any** critical vital sign/parameter (see inside back cover)
- Chemical substance or smoke burn to eye
- Severe respiratory distress (see p. 11)

Acute Triage

- Moderate respiratory distress (see p. 11)
- Visual impairment
- Fever ≥38° C rectal in infants ≤10 weeks old
- Significant trauma to eye ≤12 hours ago
- Pupil abnormalities
- Photophobia
- Fever ≥41° C oral or rectal

Urgent Triage

- Mild respiratory distress (see p. 11)
- Periorbital swelling with fever <38° C to 40.9° C oral or rectal in infants 10 to 12 weeks old
- Minor trauma to eye ≤12 hours ago
- Copious purulent eye discharge with tenderness

Nonurgent Triage

- Stable cardiorespiratory status with:
  * Visual acuity and extraocular muscles intact
  * Minor eye swelling
  * Eye discharge
  * Eye tearing
  * Eye itching
  * Conjunctivitis/iritis/uveitis
  * Fever 38° C to 40.9° C rectal or oral in children >12 weeks old

Interventions

- ◆ Complete 1° and 2° survey (p. 3)
- ◆ Assess for allergy to food, medications, insects
- ◆ Administer antipyretics for fever according to standing orders (see pp. 24 and 25)

EYE

Protocol 28 Eye Trauma

Critical Triage

- **Any** critical vital sign/parameter (see inside back cover)
- Chemical substance or smoke burn to eye
- Penetrating injury to eye
- Ruptured globe
- Eye laceration with or without hyphema

Acute Triage

- Visual impairment
- Hyphema
- Dizziness or syncopal episode
- Listless/lethargic
- Cloudy vision with flashing lights or a curtain in visual field
- Foreign body in eye
- Blunt trauma to eye or orbit ≤12 hours ago
- Clear fluid drainage from ear or nose
- Persistent vomiting
- "Blow out" orbital fracture with ↓extraocular muscle function
- Raccoon eyes (periorbital ecchymosis)
- Battle's sign (ecchymosis behind ear)
- Agonizing headache
- Pupil abnormalities

Urgent Triage

- Minor trauma to eye or orbit ≤12 hours ago
- Intermittent vomiting
- Lacerations of the periorbital area and superficial eyelid ≤12 hours ago
- Headache
- Moderate eye irritation with pain
- Inability to open eye spontaneously
- Considerable swelling or tearing of eye

Nonurgent Triage

- Stable cardiorespiratory, hydration, and neurologic status with:
  * Visual acuity and extraocular muscles intact
  * Minor injury to eye or orbit >12 hours ago *without* visual impairment
  * Minor periorbital and superficial eyelid lacerations >12 hours ago
  * Minor eye irritation with redness and/or tearing

Interventions

- ◆ Complete 1° and 2° survey (p. 3)
- ◆ ✓ GCS (see inside cover copy)
- ◆ ✓ visual acuity and extraocular movement
- ◆ ✓ pupils
- ◆ Place eye shield or soft patch over affected eye

- ◆ Keep patient seated upright in position of comfort
- ◆ Attempt to keep patient quiet and calm
- ◆ Keep NPO with traumatic eye injuries
- ◆ Keep NPO if vomiting
- ◆ Complete trauma score (see Appendix C, p. 324)

EYE

Protocol 29 Visual Disturbances

Critical Triage

- **Any** critical vital sign/parameter (see inside back cover)
- Chemical substance or smoke burn to eye
- Dextrose stick <40 mg/dl
- Stuporous, difficult to arouse

Acute Triage

- Severe headache
- Periorbital swelling *with* fever ≥38.3° C
- Listless/lethargic
- Hyphema
- Visual impairment
- Sudden loss of vision
- Persistent vomiting
- Dizziness or syncopal episode
- Cloudy vision with flashing lights or curtain in visual field
- Pupil abnormalities
- Dextrose stick 40 to 80 mg/dl
- Hx of brain tumor
- Hx of head trauma
- Hx of toxic substance ingestion
- Hx of vision disorder with acute change

Urgent Triage

- Periorbital swelling *with* fever <38.3° C
- Conjunctivitis/iritis/uveitis
- Painful headache
- Progressive loss of vision

Nonurgent Triage

- Stable cardiorespiratory and neurologic status with:
  - * Vision acuity and extraocular muscles intact
  - * Eye redness
  - * Eye discharge
  - * Eye tearing

Interventions

- ◆ Complete 1° and 2° survey (see p. 3)
- ◆ ✓ pupils
- ◆ ✓ visual acuity
- ◆ ✓ extraocular movement
- ◆ ✓ glucose via finger stick
- ◆ Place eye shield or soft patch over affected eye

EAR

Protocol 30   Earache

Critical Triage	Acute Triage
• **Any** critical vital sign/parameter (see inside back cover)	• Extreme ear pain and inconsolable irritability
• Hx of ear or head trauma *with* active clear or serosanguineous ear drainage	• Listless/lethargic
• Facial nerve paralysis or asymmetry	• Stiff neck/nuchal rigidity[†]
	• Bulging anterior fontanel
	• Hx of significant head trauma ≤12 hours ago
	• Hx of significant ear trauma ≤12 hours ago
	• Hx of significant dental trauma ≤12 hours ago
	• Fever ≥41° C oral or rectal
	• Fever ≥38° C rectal in infants ≤10 weeks old
	• Vertigo

Urgent Triage

- Foreign body in ear
- Hx of minor head trauma ≤12 hours ago
- Hx of minor ear trauma ≤12 hours ago
- Noticeable irritability and pain
- Fever ≥38° C to 40.9° C rectal in infants 10 to 12 weeks old
- Hx of minor dental trauma ≤12 hours ago

Nonurgent Triage

- Stable cardiorespiratory and neuro-logic status with:
  * Inflammation of ear canal
  * Purulent ear drainage
  * Awake and alert mental status; crying but consolable
  * Fever ≥38° C to 40.9° C oral or rectal in infants >12 weeks old
  * Toothache
  * Tugging or pulling on ear
  * Hx of minor head or ear injury >12 hours ago

Interventions

- ◆ Complete 1° and 2° survey (see p. 3)
- ◆ ✓ GCS (see inside back cover)
- ◆ Assess gross auditory function using hand clapping or ticking watch
- ◆ Administer antipyretics for fever according to standing orders (see pp. 24 and 25)

---

†Place in respiratory isolation.

EAR

Protocol 31   Ear Drainage

Critical Triage

- **Any** critical vital sign/parameter (see inside back cover)
- Stuporous, difficult to arouse
- Hx of ear or head trauma *with* active clear or serosanguineous ear drainage
- Facial nerve paralysis or asymmetry

Acute Triage

- Extreme pain and inconsolable irritability
- Listless/lethargic
- Fever ≥41° C oral or rectal
- Hx of significant head or ear trauma ≤12 hours ago *without* active ear drainage
- Fever ≥38° C rectal in infants ≤10 weeks old
- Sudden hearing loss

Urgent Triage

- Foreign body in ear
- Hx of minor head or ear trauma ≤12 hours ago *without* active ear drainage
- Fever ≥38° C to 40.9° C rectal in infants 10 to 12 weeks old
- Noticeable irritability and pain

Nonurgent Triage

- Stable cardiorespiratory and neurologic status with:
  * Inflammation of ear canal
  * Tugging or pulling on ears
  * Purulent ear drainage
  * Awake and alert mental status; crying but consolable
  * Fever ≥38° C to 40.9° C oral or rectal in children 12 weeks old
  * Hx of minor head or ear injury >12 hours ago

Interventions

- ◆ Complete 1° and 2° survey (see p. 3)
- ◆ ✓ GCS (see inside back cover)
- ◆ Assess gross auditory function using hand clapping or ticking watch
- ◆ Administer antipyretic for fever according to standing orders (see pp. 24 and 25)

EAR

Protocol 32 Ear Foreign Body

Critical Triage

- **Any** critical vital sign/parameter (see inside back cover)
- Recent Hx of head or ear trauma *with* active clear or serosanguineous ear drainage

Acute Triage

- Severe ear pain with inconsolable irritability
- Sudden hearing loss
- Penetrating injury with foreign object in ear

Urgent Triage

- Vertigo
- Foreign body in ear *with* moderate pain
- Gradual hearing loss

Nonurgent Triage

- Stable cardiorespiratory and neurologic status with foreign body in ear with mild discomfort

Interventions

- ◆ Complete 1° and 2° survey (see p. 3)
- ◆ ✓ GCS (see inside back cover)
- ◆ Assess for foreign objects (stones, beads, insects) in ear canal
- ◆ Assess gross auditory function using hand clapping or ticking watch

EAR

Protocol 33 Ear Trauma

Critical Triage	Acute Triage
• **Any** critical vital sign/parameter (see inside back cover) • Hx of severe ear or head trauma *with* active clear or serosanguineous ear drainage • Facial asymmetry or paralysis • Stuporous, difficult to arouse	• Persistent vomiting • Vertigo • Hx of significant ear or head trauma ≤12 hours ago *without* active ear drainage • Sx of moderate dehydration (see p. 11) • Sudden hearing loss • Listless/lethargic • Extreme ear pain with inconsolable irritability • Intense headache • Penetrating injury to inner ear

Urgent Triage

- Hx of minor ear or head trauma ≤12 hours ago *without* active ear drainage
- Minor ear laceration ≤12 hours ago
- Ear laceration *with* exposed cartilage
- Noticeable irritability
- Ear pain
- Painful headache
- Intermittent vomiting

Nonurgent Triage

- Stable cardiorespiratory, hydration, and neurologic status with:
  * Minor ear or head trauma >12 hours ago
  * Minor ear laceration >12 hours ago

Interventions

- ◆ Complete 1° and 2° survey (see p. 3)
- ◆ ✓ GCS (see inside back cover)
- ◆ Assess gross auditory function using hand clapping or ticking watch
- ◆ Keep NPO if vomiting
- ◆ Complete trauma score (see Appendix C, p. 324)

EAR

Protocol 34   Hearing Loss

Critical Triage	Acute Triage
• **Any** critical vital sign/parameter (see inside back cover) • Sx of severe dehydration (see p. 11)	• Orthostatic vital signs (see p. 10) • Sx of moderate dehydration (see p. 11) • Persistent vomiting • Sudden hearing loss • Intense headache • Syncopal episode • Nystagmus • Vertigo • Ataxia • Hx of diabetes mellitus • Hx of sickle cell disease • Hx of brain tumor • Hx of significant head trauma ≤12 hours ago • Hx of toxic substance ingestion • Recent Hx of menningitis • Fever ≥41° C oral or rectal

Urgent Triage

- Chronic/recurrent ear infection
- Foreign body in external ear canal
- Sx of mild dehydration (see p. 11)
- Intermittent vomiting
- Hx of minor head trauma <12 hours ago
- Progressive hearing loss
- Painful headache
- Tinnitis

Nonurgent Triage

- Stable cardiorespiratory, hydration, and neurologic status with:
  * Gross auditory function intact
  * Fever ≥38.3° C oral or rectal
  * Earache
  * Purulent drainage from ear canal
  * Hx of minor head injury >12 hours ago

Interventions

- ◆ Complete 1° and 2° survey (see p. 3)
- ◆ ✓ GCS (see inside back cover)
- ◆ Assess gross auditory function using hand clapping or ticking watch
- ◆ Assess if hearing loss is sudden or chronic

EAR

Protocol 35   Tinnitus

Critical Triage	Acute Triage
• **Any** critical vital sign/parameter (see inside back cover) • Stuporous, difficult to arouse	• Hx of significant ear or head trauma ≤12 hours ago • Hx of toxic substance ingestion ≤24 hours ago (e.g., salicylate toxicity) • Listless/lethargic • Active hallucinations, hysteria, delusions, disorganized thinking, marked disorientation[†] • Fever ≥41° C oral or rectal • Foreign body in ear *with* severe pain and inconsolable irritability

Urgent Triage

- Hx of minor ear or head trauma ≤12 hours ago
- Fever ≥38.3° C to 40.9° C oral or rectal
- Foreign body in ear *with* moderate pain and discomfort

Nonurgent Triage

- Stable cardiorespiratory and neurologic status with:
  * Recent or current ear infection
  * Hx of minor ear or head trauma >12 hours ago
  * Minor ear discomfort

Interventions

- ◆ Complete 1° and 2° survey (see p. 3)
- ◆ ✓ GCS (see inside back cover)
- ◆ Assess gross auditory function using clapping hands or ticking watch
- ◆ Administer antipyretics for fever according to standing orders (see p. 24)

---

†If patient displays unsafe behavior, notify security and place in quiet room with one-to-one supervision.

NOSE

Protocol 36 Epistaxis (Nose Bleed)

Critical Triage

- **Any** critical vital sign/parameter (see inside back cover)
- Severe frank bleeding/hemorrhage from nose or mouth
- Hx of significant facial trauma *with* severe nasal bleeding
- Hx of bleeding disorder (e.g., hemophilia)
- Hx of oncologic disorder
- Marked hypertension:
  - * SBP ≥160 if ≤10 years old
    SBP ≥170 if >10 years old
  - * DBP ≥105 if ≤10 years old
    DBP ≥110 if >10 years old

Acute Triage

- Orthostatic vital signs (see p. 10)
- Severe active bleeding from nose or mouth
- Hx of significant facial trauma *with* moderate nasal bleeding ≤12 hours ago
- Foreign body in nose *with* severe pain and irritability
- Hematemesis

Urgent Triage	Nonurgent Triage
• Moderately active nasal bleeding	• Stable cardiorespiratory status with:
• Hx of minor facial trauma ≤12 hours ago	* Minor intermittent or recurrent nasal bleeding
• Foreign body in nose *with* moderate pain and discomfort	* Hx of minor facial trauma >12 hours ago

Interventions

◆ Complete 1° and 2° survey (see p. 3)

◆ Temporary Tx of frank nasal bleeding:
  • Lean patient forward while he/she is sitting upright

• Apply direct pressure by pinching nostrils

• Place cotton roll under upper lip to compress labial artery

NOSE

Protocol **37** Nasal Drainage

Critical Triage

- **Any** critical vital sign/parameter (see inside back cover)
- Severe frank bleeding/hemorrhage from nose
- Severe respiratory distress (see p. 11)
- Hx of severe nasal or facial trauma *with* clear or serosanguineous nasal drainage
- Stuporous, difficult to arouse

Acute Triage

- Moderate respiratory distress (see p. 11)
- Severe active nasal bleeding
- Sx of moderate dehydration (see p. 11)
- Fever ≥38° C rectal in infants ≤10 weeks old
- Fever ≥41° C oral or rectal
- Stiff neck
- Listless/lethargic
- Bulging anterior fontanel
- Significant facial or orbital swelling with pain

Urgent Triage

- Mild respiratory distress (see p. 11)
- Moderately active nasal bleeding
- Fever ≥38° C to 40.9° C rectal in infants 10 to 12 weeks old

Nonurgent Triage

- Stable cardiorespiratory and hydration status with:
  * Minor intermittent nasal bleeding
  * Nasal congestion with rhinitis
  * Upper respiratory infection
  * Fever ≥38° C to 40.9° C oral or rectal in children >12 weeks old
  * Thick yellow to yellow/green purulent nasal discharge *with* facial tenderness

Interventions

- ◆ Complete 1° and 2° survey (see p. 3)
- ◆ ✓ GCS (see inside back cover)
- ◆ ✓ SpO₂
- ◆ Temporary Tx of nasal bleeding:
  - Lean patient forward while he/she is sitting upright

- Apply direct pressure by pinching nostrils
- Place cotton roll under upper lip to compress labial artery
- ◆ Administer antipyretics for fever according to standing orders (see pp. 24 and 25)

NOSE

Protocol 38 Nasal Foreign Body

Critical Triage	Acute Triage
• **Any** critical vital sign/parameter (see inside back cover) • Severe respiratory distress (see p. 11) • Severe frank bleeding/hemorrhage from nose	• Mild to moderate respiratory distress (see p. 11) • Moderately active nasal bleeding • Hematemesis • Fever ≥41° C oral or rectal

Urgent Triage	**Nonurgent Triage**
• Foreign body in nose with moderate pain and discomfort	• Stable cardiorespiratory status with:
• Minor active nasal bleeding	* Foul-smelling, purulent rhinorrhea
• Fever ≥38.3° C to 40.9° C oral or rectal	* Asymptomatic foreign body in nose

Interventions

◆ Complete 1° and 2° survey (see p. 3)

◆ Temporary Tx of frank nasal bleeding:
  • Lean patient forward while he/she is sitting upright
  • Apply direct pressure by pinching nostrils

• Place cotton roll under upper lip to compress labial artery

◆ Assess for foreign body in nose (e.g., beads, candy, stones, small toys)

NOSE

Protocol 39 Nasal Trauma

Critical Triage

- **Any** critical vital sign/parameter (see inside back cover)
- Severe respiratory distress (see p. 11)
- Penetrating injury to nose *with* clear or serosanguineous nasal drainage
- Stuporous, difficult to arouse
- Severe frank bleeding/hemorrhage from nose or mouth

Acute Triage

- Mild to moderate respiratory distress (see p. 11)
- Moderately active nasal bleeding
- Hx of significant nasal or facial trauma ≤12 hours ago
- Listless/lethargic
- Gross nasal swelling, deviation, or deformity *with* raccoon eyes (periorbital ecchymosis)
- Visual impairment
- Hyphema

Urgent Triage

- Minor active nasal bleeding
- Hx of minor nasal or facial trauma ≤12 hours ago
- Minor nasal swelling, deviation, or deformity

Nonurgent Triage

- Stable cardiorespiratory status with Hx of minor nasal trauma or facial injury >12 hours ago

Interventions

- ◆ Complete 1° and 2° survey (see p. 3)
- ◆ ✓ GCS (see inside back cover)
- ◆ Temporary Tx of frank nasal bleeding:
  - Lean patient forward while he/she is sitting upright

- Apply direct pressure by pinching nostrils
- Place cotton roll under upper lip to compress labial artery
- ◆ ✓ gross visual acuity
- ◆ Complete trauma score (see Appendix C, p. 324)

MOUTH

Protocol **40**   Dental Abscess

Critical Triage

- **Any** critical vital sign/parameter (see inside back cover)
- Unusual drooling, dysphagia, or dysphonia
- Severe respiratory distress (see p. 11)
- Sx of severe dehydration (see p. 11)

Acute Triage

- Orthostatic vital signs (see p. 10)
- Moderate respiratory distress (see p. 11)
- Sx of moderate dehydration (see p. 11)
- Fever ≥41° C oral or rectal
- Significant facial swelling *with* pain, warmth, tenderness, and erythema
- Listless/lethargic

Urgent Triage

- Mild respiratory distress (see p. 11)
- Sx of mild dehydration (see p. 11)
- Fever ≥38.3° C to 40.9° C rectal or oral
- Moderate facial swelling *with* redness, pain, and discomfort

Nonurgent Triage

- Stable cardiorespiratory and hydration status with:
  - * Halitosis
  - * Dental carry
  - * Toothache
  - * Minor facial swelling with discomfort

Interventions

- ◆ Complete 1° and 2° survey (see p. 3)
- ◆ ✓ SpO$_2$ if warranted
- ◆ ✓ GCS (see inside back cover)
- ◆ Administer antipyretics for fever according to standing orders (see pp. 24 and 25)

MOUTH

Protocol 41 Dental Trauma

Critical Triage

- **Any** critical vital sign/parameter (see inside back cover)
- Severe respiratory distress (see p. 11)
- Unusual drooling, dysphagia, or dysphonia

Acute Triage

- Mild to moderate respiratory distress (see p. 11)
- Fractured tooth
- Displaced tooth (lateral, anterior, posterior, or upward)
- Avulsed primary or secondary tooth (complete displacement of tooth from socket)
- Hx of Hemophilia
- Significant facial trauma ≤12 hours ago with obvious dental displacement or fracture

Urgent Triage

- Minor tooth injury ≤12 hours ago with loose tooth, sensory pain, or cracked tooth

Nonurgent Triage

- Stable cardiorespiratory status with minor tooth trauma >12 hours ago; dentition intact

Interventions

- ◆ Complete 1° and 2° survey (see p. 3)
- ◆ Inspect mouth for displacement and alignment of teeth
- ◆ Note any loose or fractured teeth
- ◆ Determine if injury is to primary or secondary tooth

- ◆ Avulsed permanent teeth need treatment within 30 to 60 minutes of injury:
  1. Gently wash secondary tooth
  2. Reimplant secondary tooth into socket
  3. If unable to reimplant, place tooth in milk or dental solution and save for dental consult
- ◆ Complete trauma score (see Appendix C, p. 324)

MOUTH

Protocol 42 Dysphagia

Critical Triage

- **Any** critical vital sign/parameter (see inside back cover)
- Severe respiratory distress (see p. 11)
- Sx of severe dehydration (see p. 11)
- Unusual drooling or dysphonia
- Unable to speak
- Slurred speech
- Generalized motor or sensory weakness
- Facial drooping or asymmetry
- Debilitating headache
- Stuporous, difficult to arouse
- Swelling of face, lips, or tongue

Acute Triage

- Mild to moderate respiratory distress (see p. 11)
- Fever ≥41° C oral or rectal
- Listless/lethargic
- Severe headache
- Sx of moderate dehydration (see p. 11)
- Foreign body in throat
- Significant difficulty swallowing
- Muffled voice
- Muscle stiffness of the neck

Urgent Triage

- Sx of mild dehydration (see p. 11)
- Minor difficulty swallowing
- Tonsil and adenoid surgery ≤10 days ago
- Painful headache
- Fever ≥38.3° C to 40.9° C oral or rectal
- Grossly enlarged tonsils

Nonurgent Triage

- Stable cardiorespiratory and hydration status with:
  - * Pain during swallowing
  - * Dry, scratchy, sore throat

Interventions

- ◆ Complete 1° and 2° survey (see p. 3)
- ◆ Assess respiratory and hydration status
- ◆ ✓ GCS (see inside back cover)
- ◆ ✓ motor strength and facial symmetry
- ◆ Assess for foreign body aspiration

- ◆ Assess for possible allergic reaction
- ◆ Question patient or caretaker about medications or possible drug ingestion
- ◆ Administer antipyretics for fever according to standing orders (see pp. 24 and 25).

MOUTH

Protocol 43 Mandible/Maxillary Trauma

Critical Triage

- **Any** critical vital sign/parameter (see inside back cover)
- Severe respiratory distress (see p. 11)
- Stuporous, difficult to arouse
- Multiple traumatic facial injuries
- Unusual drooling, dysphagia, dysphonia
- Clear fluid leak from nose or ear

Acute Triage

- Mild to moderate respiratory distress (see p. 11)
- Listless/lethargic
- Fractured mandible
- Fractured zygoma or facial bones
- Visual impairment
- Decreased extraocular muscle function
- Dizziness or syncopal episode
- Gross deviation of jaw or inability to open mouth
- Agonizing headache
- Significant decreased sensation to gum or cheek
- Significant mandibular or maxillary trauma ≤12 hours ago *with* loss of consciousness or persistent vomiting
- Temporomandibular joint dislocation
- Raccoon eyes (periorbital ecchymosis)
- Battle's sign (ecchymosis behind ear)
- Clear fluid leak from nose or ear

Urgent Triage	Nonurgent Triage
• Minor mandibular or maxillary trauma ≤12 hours ago	• Stable cardiorespiratory, hydration, and neurologic status with minor mandibular or maxillary trauma >12 hours ago
• Intense headache	
• Intermittent vomiting	
• Jaw clicking when opening and closing mouth	

Interventions

◆ Complete 1° and 2° survey (see p. 3)

◆ ✓ GCS (see inside back cover)

◆ ✓ pupils and extraocular muscle function

◆ Note facial symmetry of jaw movement

◆ Palpate temporomandibular joint behind ears as patient opens and closes mouth

◆ Palpate cheek and zygomatic arch for point tenderness or discontinuity

◆ Consult attending MD for radiologic studies

◆ Complete trauma score (see Appendix C, p. 324)

MOUTH

Protocol 44 Mouth Foreign Body

Critical Triage

- **Any** critical vital sign/parameter (see inside back cover)
- Severe respiratory distress (see p. 11)
- Unusual drooling, dysphagia, or dysphonia
- Unable to speak[†]

Acute Triage

- Moderate respiratory distress (see p. 11)
- Severe persistent coughing, gagging, or wretching
- Muffled voice
- Difficulty swallowing

Urgent Triage

- Mild respiratory distress (see p. 11)
- Obvious foreign body in oral cavity *without* drooling or difficult swallowing

Nonurgent Triage

- Stable cardiorespiratory status

Interventions

- ◆ Complete 1° and 2° survey (see p. 3)
- ◆ ✓ SpO$_2$

---

†If patient is unable to speak, immediately perform Heimlich maneuver to remove the obstruction.

MOUTH

Protocol 45 Mouth Lesions

Critical Triage

- **Any** critical vital sign/parameter (see inside back cover)
- Severe respiratory distress (see p. 11)
- Sx of severe dehydration (see p. 11)
- Unusual drooling, dysphagia, or dysphonia

Acute Triage

- Moderate respiratory distress (see p. 11)
- Sx of moderate dehydration (see p. 11)
- Hx of caustic substance ingestion with red burns or ulcers to oral mucosa

Urgent Triage

- Mild respiratory distress (see p. 11)
- Sx of mild dehydration (see p. 11)

Nonurgent Triage

- Stable cardiorespiratory and hydration status with:
  * Mouth sores or ulcers
  * White patches on tongue or oral mucosa
  * Painful, swollen gums

Interventions

- ◆ Complete 1° and 2° survey (p. 3)
- ◆ ✓ SpO₂
- ◆ Offer ice chips to older patients for hydration and comfort
- ◆ Offer Pedialyte or juice to infants and young patients for hydration

- ◆ For caustic ingestions, do not offer fluids and do not induce vomiting; call local poison control center (#_____-_____).

NOTE: Vesticular mouth lesions or sores in young children may indicate signs of possible sexual abuse.

MOUTH

Protocol 46 Mouth Trauma

Critical Triage

- **Any** critical vital sign/parameter (see inside back cover)
- Severe respiratory distress (see p. 11)
- Unusual drooling, dysphagia, or dysphonia
- Inability to speak
- Tracheal deviation or sudden acute swelling of neck
- Multiple traumatic facial injuries
- Stuporous, difficult to arouse

Acute Triage

- Moderate respiratory distress (see p. 11)
- Hematemesis (vomiting blood)
- Hemoptysis (coughing up blood)
- C/o foreign body in larynx when swallowing
- Severe persistent coughing, gagging, or wretching
- Oropharyngeal laceration or puncture wound to soft palate tissue
- Large tongue laceration
- Hx of hemophilia

Urgent Triage

- Minor respiratory distress (see p. 11)
- Small laceration or puncture wound to tongue ≤12 hours ago
- Laceration to gum, frenulum, or lip ≤12 hours ago
- Laceration of vermilion border of lip

Nonurgent Triage

- Stable cardiorespiratory status with laceration or puncture wound >12 hours ago to tongue, gum, or lip that does not cross vermilion border

Interventions

- ◆ Complete 1° and 2° survey (see p. 3)
- ◆ Examine neck for tracheal deviation or swelling of neck
- ◆ Inspect oropharynx for open lesions and hematomas
- ◆ Ask caretaker if patient was running with an object or stick in mouth
- ◆ Keep patient in upright position
- ◆ Offer ice chips to older children for comfort
- ◆ Complete trauma score (see Appendix C, p. 324)

MOUTH

Protocol 47 Toothache

Critical Triage

- **Any** critical vital sign/parameter (see inside back cover)
- Sx of severe dehydration (see p. 11)

Acute Triage

- Sx of moderate dehydration (see p. 11)
- Fever ≥41° C oral or rectal
- Significant facial swelling with pain, warmth, tenderness, and erythema
- Listless/lethargic

Urgent Triage

- Sx of mild dehydration (see p. 11)
- Moderate facial swelling with redness, pain, and discomfort

Nonurgent Triage

- Stable cardiorespiratory and hydration status with:
  - * Fever ≥38.3° C to 40.9° C oral or rectal
  - * Localized swelling or inflammation of gum
  - * Localized tooth pain to touch, hot, or cold
  - * Loose tooth
  - * Halitosis
  - * Minor facial swelling or discomfort

Interventions

- ◆ Complete 1° and 2° survey (see p. 3)
- ◆ Administer antipyretics for fever according to standing orders (see pp. 24 and 25)

THROAT

Protocol 48   Esophageal Foreign Body

Critical Triage

- **Any** critical vital sign/parameter (see inside back cover)
- Choking, unable to speak[†]
- Severe respiratory distress (see p. 11)
- Unusual drooling, dysphagia, or dysphonia
- Rapidly expanding swelling of neck *with* palpable subcutaneous air crepitations

Acute Triage

- Mild to moderate respiratory distress (see p. 11)
- Foreign body in throat *with* severe neck pain
- Choking episode at home *with* persistent cough, gagging, or wretching
- Hemoptysis (coughing up blood)
- Hematemesis (vomiting blood)

Urgent Triage	**Nonurgent Triage**
• Foreign body in throat *with* minimal neck pain	• Stable cardiorespiratory status with scratchy, dry, irritated throat *without* confirmed foreign body

Interventions

◆ Complete 1° and 2° survey (see p. 3)

◆ ✓ SpO$_2$

◆ Consult attending MD to obtain radiologic studies to confirm foreign body ingestion

---

†If patient is choking or unable to speak, immediately perform the Heimlich maneuver to relieve foreign body obstruction.

THROAT

Protocol 49 Neck Pain/Stiffness

Critical Triage

- **Any** critical vital sign/parameter (see inside back cover)
- Severe respiratory distress (see p. 11)
- Petechial or purpuric rash *below* nipple line with fever ≥38.3° C oral or rectal[†]
- Hx of trauma to head, neck, or back <12 hours ago *with* gross sensory or motor deficits
- Unusual drooling, dysphagia, or dysphonia

Acute Triage

- Mild to moderate respiratory distress (see p. 11)
- Listless/lethargic
- Inconsolable irritability
- Nuchal rigidity with fever ≥38.3° C oral or rectal[†]
- Severe neck pain and stiffness with fever ≥38.3° C oral or rectal
- Bulging anterior fontanel
- Vision impairment
- Dizziness or syncopal episode
- Seizure ≤12 hours ago
- Severe headache
- Petechial or purpuric rash *below* nipple line with fever <38.3° C oral or rectal[†]
- Hx of toxic substance ingestion (e.g., phenothiazines or metoclopramide)
- Hx of trauma to head, neck, or back <12 hours ago *without* sensory or motor deficits
- Sudden severe swelling of neck

Urgent Triage

- Lateral neck pain and stiffness with Hx of minor trauma ≤12 hours ago and *without* cervical pain
- Seizure >12 hours ago
- Noticeable irritability
- Intense headache
- Severe neck pain and stiffness with fever <38.3° C oral or rectal

Nonurgent Triage

- Stable cardiorespiratory and neurologic status with:
  * Sore throat
  * Lateral neck pain or stiffness *without* Hx of minor trauma
  * Minor swollen lymph nodes

Interventions

- Complete 1° and 2° survey (see p. 3)
- ✓ SpO$_2$
- Apply cervical collar to patients c/o cervical pain and notify charge nurse or attending MD

- ✓ GCS (see inside back cover)
- Question patient for Hx of trauma or ingestion
- Administer antipyretics for fever according to standing orders (see p. 24)

---

†Place patient in respiratory isolation.

THROAT

Protocol 50 Neck Trauma

Critical Triage

- **Any** critical vital sign/parameter (see inside back cover)
- Severe respiratory distress (see p. 11)
- Tracheal deviation
- Facial drooping, slurred speech
- Penetrating injury to neck or throat
- Pulsatile bleeding
- Dysphagia or dysphonia
- Hemiplegia
- Limb paresthesia
- Paralysis
- Hemiparesis/paralysis
- Generalized motor or sensory weakness
- Subcutaneous air crepitations of neck or clavicular
- Cervical pain and tenderness with light palpation or passive ROM

Acute Triage

- Mild to moderate respiratory distress (see p. 11)
- Acute epistaxis with frank bleeding
- Hemoptysis (coughing up blood)
- Hematemesis (vomiting blood)
- Severe throat pain during coughing and swallowing
- Visual impairment
- Seizure ≤12 hours ago
- Dizziness or syncopal episode
- Focal sensory or motor weakness
- Significant neck trauma ≤12 hours ago

Urgent Triage	**Nonurgent Triage**

• Throat or lateral neck pain with Hx of minor trauma <12 hours ago	• Stable cardiorespiratory and neurologic status with:
	  * Minor head or neck injury ≤12 hours ago *without* cervical pain
	  * Sore throat *without* Hx of trauma
	  * Lateral neck pain or stiffness *without* Hx of trauma

Interventions

◆ Complete 1° and 2° survey (see p. 3)

◆ ✓ SpO$_2$

◆ ✓ GCS (see inside back cover)

◆ Examine throat for tracheal deviation

◆ Palpate clavicular area and neck for subcutaneous air crepitations

◆ Apply cervical collar to patients c/o cervical pain and notify charge nurse or attending MD

◆ Apply NSS pressure dressing to open wounds

◆ Complete trauma score (see Appendix C, p. 324)

THROAT

Protocol **51** Sore Throat

Critical Triage

- **Any** critical vital sign/parameter (see inside back cover)
- Severe respiratory distress (see p. 11)
- Unusual drooling, dysphagia, or dysphonia
- Sx of severe dehydration (see p. 11)
- Unable to speak

Acute Triage

- Orthostatic vital signs (see p. 10)
- Moderate respiratory distress (see p. 11)
- Sx of moderate dehydration (see p. 11)
- Significant difficulty swallowing
- Muffled voice
- Listless/lethargic
- Tonsil and adenoid surgery <10 days ago with peritonsilar bleeding
- Fever ≥41° C oral or rectal
- Foreign body in throat with severe neck pain

Urgent Triage

- Mild respiratory distress (see p. 11)
- Sx of mild dehydration (see p. 11)
- Grossly enlarged, painful tonsils
- Foreign body in throat with minimal neck pain

Nonurgent Triage

- Stable cardiorespiratory and hydration status with:
  * Fever ≥38.3° C to 40.9° C oral or rectal
  * Able to swallow; no drooling
  * Inflamed, red, sore pharynx with possible exudate
  * Painful to swallow
  * Scratchy, dry, irritated throat

Interventions

- Complete 1° and 2° survey (see p. 3)
- ✓ GCS (see inside cover copy)
- ✓ SpO_2
- Administer antipyretics for fever according to standing orders (see p. 24)

- Obtain throat culture according to protocol
- Question caretaker about possible foreign body aspiration at home

NOTE: If patient is drooling or has significant respiratory distress, do **not** obtain throat culture or attempt to visualize the posterior pharynx during triage—this may cause respiratory compromise and arrest.

THROAT

Protocol 52   Swollen Glands

Critical Triage

- **Any** critical vital sign/parameter (see inside back cover)
- Severe respiratory distress (see p. 11)
- Sx of severe dehydration (see p. 11)
- Unusual drooling, dysphagia, or dysphonia

Acute Triage

- Orthostatic vital signs (see p. 10)
- Moderate respiratory distress (see p. 11)
- Sx of moderate dehydration (see p. 11)
- Fever >41° C oral or rectal
- Fever ≥38° C rectal in infants ≤10 weeks old
- Listless/lethargic
- Significant swelling of lateral neck area with warmth, tenderness, and erythema
- Muffled voice

Urgent Triage

- Mild respiratory distress (see p. 11)
- Sx of mild dehydration (see p. 11)
- Fever ≥38° C to 40.9° C rectal or oral in infants 10 to 12 weeks old
- Grossly enlarged, painful tonsils

Nonurgent Triage

- Stable cardiorespiratory and hydration status with:
  * Fever ≥38° C to 40.9° C oral or rectal in children >12 weeks old
  * Minor upper respiratory tract infection
  * Earache
  * Dry, scratchy, sore throat
  * Large, warm, firm, red node tender to palpation
  * Slow growing, painless, firm node in neck

Interventions

- ◆ Complete 1° and 2° survey (see p. 3)
- ◆ ✓ SpO_2
- ◆ Administer antipyretics for fever according to standing orders (see pp. 24 and 25)

GASTROINTESTINAL

Protocol 53 Abdominal Pain (Gastrointestinal)

Critical Triage	Acute Triage

Critical Triage

- **Any** critical vital sign/parameter (see inside back cover)
- Stuporous, difficult to arouse
- Severe respiratory distress (see p. 11)
- Agonizing abdominal pain

Acute Triage

- Orthostatic vital signs (see p. 10)
- Sx of moderate dehydration (see p. 11)
- Listless/lethargic
- Severe abdominal pain
- Involuntary abdominal guarding with rebound tenderness
- Absent bowel sounds
- Markedly distended or rigid abdomen
- Hematuria
- Purpura
- Currant jelly stools
- Frank blood in stools or rectum
- Vomiting frank blood, bilious or coffee ground fluid
- Severe jaundice
- Marked pallor
- Irreducible (incarcerated) hernia
- Hx of significant abdominal trauma <12 hours ago
- Hx of sickle cell disease
- Hx of inflammatory bowel disease
- Referred *left* shoulder pain
- Fever ≥41° C oral or rectal

Urgent Triage

- Sx of mild dehydration (see p. 11)
- Irritable or restless
- Mild tachycardia
- Moderate abdominal pain
- Decreased bowel sounds
- Flank tenderness
- Abdominal pain with jumping or hopping without Hx of trauma
- Persistent vomiting
- Persistent diarrhea
- Mucous, foul smelling, frothy stools
- Constipated ≥5 days
- Blood streaks in stools
- Hx of minor abdominal injury ≤12 hours ago
- Moderate abdominal distension
- Fever ≥38.3° C oral or rectal with right lower quadrant (RLQ) pain

Nonurgent Triage

- Stable cardiorespiratory and hydration status with:
  * Minor abdominal injury >12 hours ago
  * Minor abdominal pain or stomach-ache
  * Colic
  * ↑stool frequency
  * Flatus
  * Menstrual cramps
  * Dysuria
  * Constipated ≤5 days
  * Loose stools with scant dark blood flecks
  * Mild abdominal distension

Interventions

- Complete 1° and 2° survey (see p. 3)
- Ask patient to jump or hop to check for signs of abdominal pain consistent with peritoneal irritation
- Obtain urine pregnancy screen on any potentially pregnant patient

- Obtain urinalysis (U/A) on patient c/o dysuria
- Guaiac stool for presence of blood
- Administer antipyretic for fever according to standing orders (see pp. 24 and 25)

GASTROINTESTINAL

Protocol 54 Abdominal Trauma

Critical Triage	**Acute Triage**
• **Any** critical vital sign/parameter (see inside back cover)	• Orthostatic vital signs (see p. 10)
• Multiple traumatic injuries (see p. 11)	• Listless/lethargic
• Severe respiratory distress (see p. 11)	• Significant pallor or jaundice
• Marked pallor of mucous membranes	• Dizziness or syncopal episode
• Penetrating abdominal injury	• Seizure ≤12 hours ago
• Agonizing abdominal pain	• Distended painful, rigid abdomen
	• Bilious vomiting
	• Hematemesis
	• Hematuria
	• Frank rectal bleeding
	• +hop test with peritoneal irritation
	• Absent bowel sounds
	• Referred *left* shoulder pain (questionable splenic injury)
	• Hx of blunt trauma to abdomen ≤12 hours ago
	• Severe abdominal pain
	• Involuntary abdominal guarding or rebound tenderness

Urgent Triage

- Minor abdominal injury ≤12 hours ago
- Seizure >12 hours ago
- Persistent vomiting
- Blood streaks in stool

Nonurgent Triage

- Stable cardiorespiratory and hydration status with:
  * Minor abdominal injury >12 hours ago
  * Awake, alert, cooperative mental status
  * Occasional vomiting

Interventions

- Complete 1° and 2° survey (see p. 3)
- ✓ GCS (see inside back cover)
- Ask patient to hop or jump to check for signs of abdominal pain consistent with peritoneal irritation

- Guaiac stools for presence of blood
- Keep NPO if vomiting
- Complete trauma score (see Appendix C, p. 324)

GASTROINTESTINAL

Protocol **55** Constipation

Critical Triage	Acute Triage

Critical Triage

- **Any** critical vital sign/parameter (see inside back cover)
- Severe respiratory distress (see p. 11)
- Sx of severe dehydration (see p. 11)
- Stuporous, difficult to arouse

Acute Triage

- Moderate respiratory distress (see p. 11)
- Sx of moderate dehydration (see p. 11)
- Listless/lethargic
- Markedly distended, rigid abdomen
- +hop test with peritoneal irritation
- Vomiting brown or bilious fluid
- Absent bowel sounds
- Severe abdominal pain
- Hx of Hirschsprung's disease

Urgent Triage

- Mild respiratory distress (see p. 11)
- Sx of mild dehydration (see p. 11)
- Moderate abdominal pain/discomfort
- No passage of stool ≥5 days
- Moderate abdominal distension

Nonurgent Triage

- Stable cardiorespiratory and hydration status with:
  * ↓ frequency of passage of stool
  * Abdomen slightly distended but soft and nontender
  * Mild abdominal distension

Interventions

- ◆ Complete 1° and 2° survey (see p. 3)
- ◆ ✓ GCS (see inside back cover)
- ◆ Inspect abdomen for size and shape
- ◆ Palpate abdomen for tenderness and masses

- ◆ Ask patient to hop or jump to ✓ for signs of abdominal pain consistent with peritoneal irritation
- ◆ Inquire about cathartic use at home

GASTROINTESTINAL

Protocol 56 Diarrhea

Critical Triage	Acute Triage

Critical Triage

- **Any** critical vital sign/parameter (see inside back cover)
- Severe respiratory distress (see p. 11)
- Sx of severe dehydration (see p. 11)
- Stuporous, difficult to arouse

Acute Triage

- Orthostatic vital signs (see p. 10)
- Sx of moderate dehydration (see p. 11)
- Listless/lethargic
- Extreme unconsolable irritability
- Fever ≥41° C oral or rectal
- Fever ≥38° C rectal in infants ≤10 weeks old
- Severe crampy abdominal pain
- Hx of inflammatory bowel disease (flare-up)
- Passage of bloody, currant jelly stool
- Frank bloody diarrhea
- Hematuria
- Purpura
- Markedly distended, rigid abdomen
- Severe abdominal pain

Urgent Triage

- Sx of mild dehydration (see p. 11)
- Fever ≥38° C to 40.9° C rectal in infants 10 to 12 weeks old
- Noticeable irritability but consolable
- Bloody streaks in stool
- Moderate abdominal pain or cramping

Nonurgent Triage

- Stable cardiorespiratory and hydration status with:
  - * Loose, watery stools with increased frequency
  - * Fever ≥38° C to 40.9° C in infants ≥12 weeks old
  - * Stools with scant, dark blood flecks
  - * Mild abdominal discomfort or cramping

Interventions

- ◆ Complete 1° and 2° survey (see p. 3)
- ◆ ✓ GCS (see inside back cover)
- ◆ Assess character of stool for color, consistency, and amount of diarrhea
- ◆ Guaiac stool for presence of blood

- ◆ Administer antipyretics for fever according to standing orders (see pp. 24 and 25)
- ◆ Keep NPO for *all* acute triage conditions

GASTROINTESTINAL

Protocol 57 Feeding Tube Problems (GT, JT, NG, OG†)

Critical Triage

- **Any** critical vital sign/parameter (see inside back cover)
- Stuporous, difficult to arouse
- Sx of severe dehydration (see p. 11)

Acute Triage

- Orthostatic vital signs (see p. 10)
- Sx of moderate dehydration (see p. 11)
- Listless/lethargic
- Dextrose stick 40 to 80 mg/dl
- Gastric tube replacement

---

†*GT*, gastrotomy tube; *JT*, jejunostomy tube; *NG*, nasogastric tube; *OG*, oral gastric tube.

Urgent Triage

- Sx of mild dehydration (see p. 11)
- Hx of gastrointestinal disorder
- Hx of metabolic disorder
- Clogged gastric tube
- Broken gastric tube (tube remains in stoma)
- NG or OG tube replacement

Nonurgent Triage

- None
- Triage other Sx

Interventions

- ◆ Complete 1° and 2° survey (see p. 3)
- ◆ ✓ GCS (see inside back cover)
- ◆ ✓ for signs of dehydration (see p. 11)
- ◆ ✓ glucose via finger stick

NOTE: Gastric tubes that are out of stoma need to be replaced in a timely fashion because stoma may close.

GASTROINTESTINAL

Protocol 58 Gastrointestinal Bleeding

Critical Triage	Acute Triage
• **Any** critical vital sign/parameter (see inside back cover) • Sx of severe dehydration (see p. 11) • Profuse frank gastrointestinal (GI) bleeding/hemorrhaging • Stuporous, difficult to arouse	• Orthostatic vital signs (see p. 10) • Sx of moderate dehydration (see p. 11) • Marked pallor • Vomiting bright red blood • Severe abdominal pain • Vomiting coffee ground fluid • Hx of bleeding disorder • Hx of liver disease • Hx of swallowing foreign body

Urgent Triage	Nonurgent Triage
• Sx of mild dehydration (see p. 11)	• Stable cardiorespiratory and hydration status with:
• Vomiting coffee ground fluid	* Vomiting fluid with scant flecks of old dark blood
• Moderate abdominal cramping or discomfort	* Vomiting red fluid, guaiac negative
• Reliable Hx of vomiting of blood at home *without* active bleeding	

Interventions

◆ Complete 1° and 2° survey (see p. 3)	◆ Ask caretaker or patient if patient recently ingested fluid or food with red dye, such as gelatin, frozen juice bar, water, ice or punch
◆ Keep patient seated in upright position	
◆ Guaiac emesis to check for presence of blood	

GASTROINTESTINAL

Protocol 59 Nausea

Critical Triage

- **Any** critical vital sign/parameter (see inside back cover)
- Sx of severe dehydration (see p. 11)
- Stuporous, difficult to arouse

Acute Triage

- Orthostatic vital signs (see p. 10)
- Sx of moderate dehydration (see p. 11)
- Listless/lethargic
- Hx of toxic substance ingestion ≤12 hours ago
- Dextrose stick 40 to 80 mg/dl
- Severe abdominal pain

Urgent Triage

- Sx of mild dehydration (see p. 11)
- Hx of toxic substance ingestion >12 hours ago
- Mild to moderate abdominal pain
- Chronic morning nausea and vomiting

Nonurgent Triage

- Stable cardiorespiratory and hydration status with:
  * Missed or late menses in adolescent girls
  * Intermittent nausea

Interventions

- ◆ Complete 1° and 2° survey (see p. 3)
- ◆ ✓ GCS (see inside back cover)
- ◆ ✓ glucose via finger stick
- ◆ Obtain urine pregnancy screen for adolescent girls c/o nausea and late menses according to standing orders (see p. 27)

GASTROINTESTINAL

Protocol 60 Rectal Bleeding

Critical Triage

- **Any** critical vital sign/parameter (see inside back cover)
- Sx of severe dehydration (see p. 11)
- Profuse frank rectal bleeding/hemorrhaging
- Stuporous, difficult to arouse

Acute Triage

- Orthostatic vital signs (see p. 10)
- Listless/lethargic
- Sx of moderate dehydration (see p. 11)
- Marked pallor
- Active rectal bleeding of bright red blood
- Severe abdominal pain
- Rigid, distended, tender abdomen
- Currant jelly stool
- Purpura
- Hematuria
- Hx of bleeding disorder
- Hx of inflammatory bowel disease

Urgent Triage

- Sx of mild dehydration (see p. 11)
- Moderate abdominal cramping or discomfort
- Bloody streaks of diarrhea
- Dark black stool
- Reliable Hx of rectal bleeding at home *without* active bleeding
- Rectal prolapse

Nonurgent Triage

- Stable cardiorespiratory and hydration status with:
  * Stools with scant dark blood flecks
  * Hemorrhoids or rectal polyps
  * Stools with red coloring, guaiac negative
  * Obvious anal fissure
  * Excoriated rectal area

Interventions

- ◆ Complete 1° and 2° survey (see p. 3)
- ◆ Guaiac stools to check for presence of blood
- ◆ Ask caretaker or patient if patient recently ingested fluid or foods

containing red dye; such as gelatin, frozen juice bar, water-ice, or punch
- ◆ Keep NPO

GASTROINTESTINAL

Protocol 61 Rectal Foreign Body

Critical Triage	Acute Triage

Critical Triage

- **Any** critical vital sign/parameter (see inside back cover)
- Profuse frank bleeding/hemorrhaging from rectum
- Stuporous, difficult to arouse

Acute Triage

- Orthostatic vital signs (see p. 10)
- Fever ≥41° C oral
- Moderately active rectal bleeding
- Listless/lethargic
- Intense rectal or abdominal bleeding
- Rigid, distended, tender abdomen
- Involuntary abdominal guarding; rebound tenderness
- Rectal laceration ≤12 hours ago

Urgent Triage

- Considerable rectal or abdominal pain
- Fever ≥38.3° C to 40.9° C oral
- Minor rectal laceration >12 hours ago
- Minor rectal bleeding

Nonurgent Triage

- Stable cardiorespiratory status with asymptomatic rectal foreign body

Interventions

- ◆ Complete 1° and 2° survey (see p. 3)
- ◆ ✓ GCS (see inside back cover)
- ◆ Administer antipyretics for fever according to standing orders (see pp. 24 and 25)
- ◆ Have patient jump or hop to assess for signs of peritoneal irritation

GASTROINTESTINAL

Protocol 62 Vomiting

Critical Triage	Acute Triage
• **Any** critical vital sign/parameter (see inside back cover)	• Orthostatic vital signs (see p. 10)
• Sx of severe dehydration (see p. 11)	• Sx of moderate dehydration (see p. 11)
• Stuporous, difficult to arouse	• Profuse vomiting
• Profuse vomiting of frank blood	• Listless/lethargic
	• Hematemesis
	• Bilious vomiting
	• Vomiting stool or coffee ground fluid
	• Severe abdominal pain
	• Markedly distended, rigid abdomen
	• Severe abdominal pain
	• Involuntary abdominal guarding with rebound tenderness
	• Fever ≥41° C oral or rectal
	• Fever ≥38° C rectal in infants ≤10 weeks old
	• Hx of diabetes
	• Hx of head trauma
	• Hx of toxic substance ingestion
	• Hx of metabolic disorder
	• Hx of ventroperitoneal shunt

Urgent Triage

- Sx of mild dehydration (see p. 11)
- Fever ≥38.3° C to 40.9° C rectal in infants 10 to 12 weeks old
- Persistent vomiting
- Moderate abdominal pain or discomfort
- Chronic morning nausea and vomiting

Nonurgent Triage

- Stable cardiorespiratory and hydration status with:
  * Occasional vomiting
  * "Spitting up" food or fluids
  * Fever ≥38° c to 40.9° C oral or rectal in infants >12 weeks old

Interventions

- Complete 1° and 2° survey (see p. 3)
- ✓ GCS (see inside back cover)
- Assess emesis for color, consistency, and amount
- Guaiac emesis for blood
- Ask patient to hop or jump to check for signs of abdominal pain consistent with peritoneal irritation
- Administer antipyretics for fever according to protocols (see pp. 260 and 262)
- Keep NPO

GYNECOLOGIC

Protocol 63 Abdominal Pain (Gynecologic)

Critical Triage

- **Any** critical vital sign/parameter (see inside back cover)
- Pregnant with impending delivery
- Agonizing abdominal pain

Acute Triage

- Sexually active female adolescent with severe abdominal pain
- Involuntary abdominal guarding or rebound tenderness
- Markedly distended, rigid abdomen
- Absent bowel sounds
- Pregnant female adolescent with vaginal bleeding
- Fever ≥41° C oral
- Profuse vomiting
- Frank vaginal bleeding

Urgent Triage	Nonurgent Triage
• Sexually active female adolescent with moderate abdominal pain	• Stable cardiorespiratory and hydration status with:
• Persistent vomiting	* Dysuria
• Flank tenderness	* Menstrual cramps
• Purulent, foul-smelling vaginal discharge	* Increased vaginal discharge
• Abnormally heavy vaginal bleeding	* White-yellow, thick vaginal discharge
• Fever ≥38.3° C to 40.9° C oral	* Minor abdominal discomfort
	* Minor vaginal bleeding

Interventions

◆ Complete 1° and 2° survey (see p. 3)

◆ Determine date of last menstrual period

◆ Obtain urine pregnancy test for any potentially pregnant patient

◆ Obtain routine U/A if c/o dysuria

◆ Ask patient to jump or hop to assess for signs of abdominal pain consistent with peritoneal irritation

◆ Administer antipyretics for fever according to standing orders (see pp. 24 and 25)

GYNECOLOGIC

Protocol **64** Menstrual Cramps

Critical Triage	Acute Triage
• **Any** critical vital sign/parameter (see inside back cover) • Agonizing abdominal pain	• Fever ≥41° C oral • Severe lower abdominal pain • Rigid abdomen • Involuntary abdominal guarding with rebound tenderness • Severe headache • Profuse vomiting or diarrhea • Severe headache

Urgent Triage

- Considerable lower abdominal pain with fever ≥38.3° C to 40.9° C oral
- Considerable abdominal pain with hopping or jumping (+hop test)
- Persistent vomiting or diarrhea
- Palpable pelvic mass
- Moderately painful headache

Nonurgent Triage

- Stable cardiorespiratory and hydration status with:
  - * Mild lower abdominal discomfort or cramping
  - * Mild headache
  - * Backache
  - * Leg pain
  - * Mild nausea, vomiting, or diarrhea

Interventions

- ◆ Complete 1° and 2° survey (see p. 3)
- ◆ Determine date of last menstrual period
- ◆ Ask patient to jump or hop to assess for signs of abdominal pain

consistent with peritoneal irritation
- ◆ Administer antipyretics for fever according to standing orders (see pp. 24 and 25)

GYNECOLOGIC

Protocol 65 Teenage Pregnancy

Critical Triage

- **Any** critical vital sign/parameter (see inside back cover)
- Pregnant adolescent with impending delivery
- Profuse frank vaginal bleeding/hemorrhaging

Acute Triage

- Orthostatic vital signs (see p. 10)
- Active, bright red vaginal bleeding
- Faint or lightheaded
- Dextrose stick 40 to 80 mg/dl
- Active contractions
- Severe lower abdominal or back pain

Urgent Triage

- Hx of syncopal episode before arrival to ER
- Moderate lower abdominal pain
- Minor vaginal bleeding

Nonurgent Triage

- Stable cardiorespiratory status with positive pregnancy test (serum or urine) asymptomatic[†]

Interventions

- ◆ Complete 1° and 2° survey (see p. 3)
- ◆ Determine last menstrual period and gestational age of fetus
- ◆ Obtain urine pregnancy test as per standing orders (see p. 27) if pregnancy is unconfirmed
- ◆ Obtain glucose via finger stick

[†]If patient has positive pregnancy test and is stable, refer to adult OB/GYN facility for care.

GYNECOLOGIC

Protocol 66 Vaginal Bleeding

Critical Triage

- **Any** critical vital sign/parameter (see inside back cover)
- Profuse frank vaginal bleeding/hemorrhaging
- Penetrating traumatic vaginal injury
- Pregnant patient with impending delivery

Acute Triage

- Orthostatic vital signs (see p. 10)
- Severe active vaginal bleeding (bright red blood)
- Hx of significant vaginal trauma ≤12 hours ago
- Severe lower abdominal pain
- Pregnant adolescent with vaginal bleeding
- Hx of syncopal episode
- Marked pallor
- Petechiae or purpura rash

Urgent Triage

- Moderately active vaginal bleeding >9 days
- Moderate abdominal pain or discomfort
- Vaginal bleeding *before* menarche
- Hx of minor vaginal trauma 12 to 24 hours ago
- Hx of possible sexual assault
- Pelvic mass
- Urethral prolapse

Nonurgent Triage

- Stable cardiorespiratory status with:
  * Minor vaginal bleeding or discharge
  * Prolonged menses
  * Hx of minor vaginal injury >24 hours ago
  * Genital warts
  * Minor abdominal discomfort
  * Hx of vaginal bleeding at home

Interventions

- ◆ Complete 1° and 2° survey (see p. 3)
- ◆ Determine if patient is premenarchal or menarchal (check breast development, pubic hair)
- ◆ Assess vaginal bleeding for amount (pads per day/hour), color, consistency, and duration
- ◆ Determine last menstrual period
- ◆ Obtain urine pregnancy test according to standing orders (see p. 27) on potentially pregnant patients

NOTE: Vaginal bleeding in the premenarchal female may indicate possible sexual assault.

GYNECOLOGIC

Protocol **67**   Vaginal Discharge

Critical Triage

- **Any** critical vital sign/parameter (see inside back cover)

Acute Triage

- Pregnant with copious clear vaginal secretions
- Fever ≥41° C oral or rectal
- Severe lower abdominal pain
- Fever ≥38.3° C rectal in infants ≤10 weeks old

Urgent Triage

- Fever ≥38.3° C to 40.9° C rectal in infants 10 to 12 weeks old
- Fever ≥38.3° C to 40.9° C in older female adolescent with moderate abdominal pain
- Flank tenderness
- Purulent, foul-smelling vaginal discharge with moderate abdominal pain
- Hx of possible sexual assault
- Painful vaginal discharge in prepubertal female patients

Nonurgent Triage

- Stable cardiorespiratory status with:
  * Asymptomatic vaginal discharge in infants ≤4 weeks old
  * Asymptomatic vaginal discharge in pubertal females
  * Dysuria
  * Vaginal irritation and discomfort
  * White-yellow, thick vaginal secretions
  * Vaginal itching

Interventions

- ◆ Complete 1° and 2° survey (see p. 3)
- ◆ Assess vaginal discharge for color, amount, odor, and duration
- ◆ Administer antipyretics for fever according to standing orders (see pp. 24 and 25)

NOTE: Healthy infants >4 weeks old and prepubertal females do not normally have liquid vaginal secretions; presence of vaginal discharge may indicate sexual abuse.

GYNECOLOGIC

Protocol 68 Vaginal Foreign Body

Critical Triage

- **Any** critical vital sign/parameter (see inside back cover)
- Profuse frank bleeding/hemorrhaging from vagina

Acute Triage

- Moderately active vaginal bleeding
- Intense genital or abdominal pain
- Fever ≥41° C oral
- Vaginal laceration ≤12 hours ago

Urgent Triage

- Genital pain
- Fever ≥38.3° C to 40.9° C oral
- Purulent, foul-smelling vaginal discharge
- Minor vaginal laceration >12 hours ago
- Minor active vaginal bleeding

Nonurgent Triage

- Stable cardiorespiratory status with:
  * Dysuria
  * Minor genital discomfort
  * Asymptomatic vaginal foreign body
  * Increased vaginal discharge in pubertal female patients
  * Scant pink vaginal discharge

Interventions

- ◆ Complete 1° and 2° survey (see p. 3)
- ◆ Administer antipyretics for fever according to standing orders (see pp. 24 and 25)

GENITALIA

Protocol 69   Genital Itching

Critical Triage	Acute Triage
• **Any** critical vital sign/parameter (see inside back cover)	• Fever ≥41° C oral • Severe abdominal or genital pain with involuntary guarding and rebound tenderness

Urgent Triage	**Nonurgent Triage**
• Hx of sexual abuse	• Stable cardiorespiratory and hydration status with:
• Considerable genital pain and irritation	* Minor genital discomfort
• Fever ≥38.3° C to 40.9° C oral	* Rectal or genital pruritus
• Flank tenderness	* Pinworms
• Pyuria	* Dysuria
• Purulent, foul-smelling penile or vaginal discharge	• Penile swelling
	• White-yellow-green vaginal or penile discharge
	• Vaginal or penile irritation

Interventions

◆ Complete 1° and 2° survey (see p. 3)

◆ Administer antipyretics for fever according to standing orders (see pp. 24 and 25)

GENITALIA

Protocol 70   Genital Lesions

Critical Triage

- **Any** critical vital sign/parameter (see inside back cover)

Acute Triage

- Fever ≥41° C oral
- Severe abdominal or genital pain with involuntary guarding and rebound tenderness

Urgent Triage

- Hx of sexual abuse
- Fever ≥38.3° C to 40.9° C oral
- Purulent, foul-smelling penile or vaginal discharge
- Flank tenderness
- Pyuria
- Painful, swollen, fluctuant mass of labia minora

Nonurgent Triage

- Stable cardiorespiratory and hydration status with:
  * Minor genital discomfort
  * Minor genital irritation or ulcers
  * Penile swelling
  * Dysuria
  * Asymptomatic genital warts or ulcers
  * Scant bloody vaginal discharge

Interventions

- ◆ Complete 1° and 2° survey (see p. 3)
- ◆ Administer antipyretics for fever according to standing orders (see pp. 24 and 25)

NOTE: Genital warts and ulcers are very rare in the prepubertal child and warrants further investigation for possible sexual abuse.

GENITALIA

Protocol 71 Genital Trauma

Critical Triage

- **Any** critical vital sign/parameter (see inside back cover)
- Profuse frank vaginal or penile bleeding/hemorrhaging
- Penetrating genitourinary injury

Acute Triage

- Hx of significant vaginal, rectal, scrotal, or penile trauma ≤12 hours ago
- Sudden dark blue discoloration of the testes
- Intense abdominal/genital pain with involuntary guarding and rebound tenderness
- Considerable active vaginal, rectal, or penile bleeding
- Vaginal, penile, or rectal laceration ≤12 hours ago
- Inability to void caused by pain and edema
- Significant painful scrotal swelling

Urgent Triage

- Hx of minor vaginal, rectal, scrotal, or penile trauma ≤12 hours ago
- Moderate abdominal pain and discomfort
- Vaginal, rectal, penile, or scrotal laceration >12 hours ago
- Moderately active vaginal, penile, or rectal bleeding
- Hematuria
- Minor zipper entrapment of the penis

Nonurgent Triage

- Stable cardiorespiratory status with:
  * Hx of minor vaginal, rectal, scrotal, or penile trauma >12 hours ago
  * Minor genital pain or discomfort
  * Minor genital swelling

Interventions

- ◆ Complete 1° and 2° survey (see p. 3)
- ◆ Inspect genital area for hematoma, bleeding, swelling, and lacerations
- ◆ Determine if Hx is consistent with the mechanism of injury

- ◆ Apply mineral oil to skin to relieve zipper entrapment injuries
- ◆ Complete trauma score (see Appendix C, p. 324)

NOTE: Genital trauma in young children with inconsistent Hx and mechanism of injury warrants investigation for possible sexual abuse.

GENITALIA

Protocol 72 Hernia

Critical Triage

- **Any** critical vital sign/parameter (see inside back cover)

Acute Triage

- Listless/lethargic
- Inconsolable irritability
- Firm, irreducible scrotal or inguinal hernia
- Significant lower abdominal or genital pain
- Marked abdominal distension
- Profuse vomiting
- Involuntary abdominal guarding with rebound tenderness
- Dark blue discoloration of testis
- Fever ≥38° C rectal in infants ≤10 weeks old
- Fever ≥41° C oral or rectal

Urgent Triage

- *Painful* intermittent swelling of inguinal canal or scrotal area when crying or straining
- Intermittent vomiting
- Moderate lower abdominal or genital pain
- Noticeable irritability
- Fever ≥38° C to 40.9° C rectal in infants 10 to 12 weeks old

Nonurgent Triage

- Stable cardiorespiratory and hydration status with:
  * *Painless* intermittent swelling of inguinal canal or scrotal area when crying or straining
  * Fever ≥38° C to 40.9° C oral or rectal in infants >12 weeks old

Interventions

- ◆ Complete 1° and 2° survey (see p. 3)
- ◆ Assess hernia for location, size, firmness, and reducibility
- ◆ Keep NPO if vomiting
- ◆ Administer antipyretics for fever according to standing orders (see pp. 24 and 25)

GENITALIA

Protocol 73 Penile Swelling

Critical Triage

- **Any** critical vital sign/parameter (see inside back cover)

Acute Triage

- Significant genital trauma ≤12 hours ago
- Priapism with Hx of sickle cell disease

Urgent Triage

- Considerable difficulty in voiding caused by excessive penile inflammation
- Minor genital trauma ≤12 hours ago
- Moderately painful penile edema
- Zipper entrapment of penis

Nonurgent Triage

- Stable cardiorespiratory status with:
  * Minor inflammation of glans of penis
  * Minor genital injury >12 hours ago
  * Minor redness, inflammation, and tenderness of the penis
  * Local insect bite
  * Dysuria
  * Irritated red rash in diaper area

Interventions

- ◆ Complete 1° and 2° survey (see p. 3)
- ◆ Inspect penis for evidence of trauma, degree of swelling, irritation, tenderness, and ability to void
- ◆ Apply mineral oil to skin of penis to relieve zipper entrapment injuries

GENITALIA

Protocol 74 Scrotal Pain/Swelling

Critical Triage

- **Any** critical vital sign/parameter (see inside back cover)

Acute Triage

- Orthostatic vital signs (see p. 10)
- Sx of moderate dehydration (see p. 11)
- Severe scrotal pain
- Acute scrotal swelling with severe pain
- Sudden dark discoloration of testis
- Persistent vomiting
- Intense lower abdominal/genital pain
- Significant scrotal trauma ≤12 hours ago

Urgent Triage

- Sx of mild dehydration (see p. 11)
- Intermittent vomiting
- Minor scrotal trauma ≤12 hours ago
- Gradual swelling and tenderness of the testis
- Painful intermittent swelling of scrotal area with crying or straining

Nonurgent Triage

- Stable cardiorespiratory status with:
  * Dysuria
  * Urinary frequency and urgency
  * Minor scrotal injury >12 hours ago
  * Painless scrotal swelling not associated with trauma or crying

Interventions

- ◆ Complete 1° and 2° survey (see p. 3)
- ◆ Inspect testis for swelling or discoloration
- ◆ Ask patient to rate scrotal pain on scale of 1 (none) to 10 (severe)
- ◆ Patients with painful scrotal swelling should remain NPO

GENITALIA

Protocol 75 Urethral Discharge

Critical Triage

- **Any** critical vital sign/parameter (see inside back cover)

Acute Triage

- Fever ≥41° C oral
- Severe abdominal/flank pain with involuntary guarding and rebound tenderness
- Inability to void

Urgent Triage

- Considerable difficulty voiding
- Considerable abdominal/flank pain
- Fever ≥38.3° C to 40.9° C oral

Nonurgent Triage

- Stable cardiorespiratory status with:
  * Dysuria
  * Foul-smelling, cloudy urine
  * White-yellow-green penile discharge
  * Pruritis

Interventions

- ◆ Complete 1° and 2° survey (see p. 3)
- ◆ Assess urethral discharge for amount, color, odor, pain, duration, and difficulty
- ◆ Administer antipyretics for fever according to standing orders (see pp. 24 and 25)

GENITALIA

Protocol 76 Urethral Foreign Body

Critical Triage	Acute Triage
• **Any** critical vital sign/parameter (see inside back cover) • Profuse frank bleeding/hemorrhaging from penile area	• Moderately active penile bleeding • Intense genital or abdominal pain • Inability to void • Fever ≥41° C oral • Penile laceration <12 hours ago

Urgent Triage

- Considerable genital pain
- Fever ≥38.3° C to 40.9° C oral
- Purulent, foul-smelling penile discharge
- Penile laceration >12 hours ago
- Minor active penile bleeding
- Considerable difficulty voiding

Nonurgent Triage

- Stable cardiorespiratory status with:
  * Dysuria
  * Minor genital discomfort
  * Asymptomatic urethral foreign body

Interventions

- ◆ Complete 1° and 2° survey (see p. 3)
- ◆ Administer antipyretics for fever according to standing orders (see pp. 24 and 25)

UROLOGIC/RENAL

Protocol 77 Decreased Urination

Critical Triage

- **Any** critical vital sign/parameter (see inside back cover)
- Sx of severe dehydration (see p. 11)
- Stuporous, difficult to arouse
- Marked hypertension:
  - * SBP ≥160 if ≤10 years old
    SBP ≥170 if >10 years old
  - * DBP ≥105 if ≤10 years old
    DBP ≥110 if >10 years old

Acute Triage

- Orthostatic vital signs (see p. 10)
- Sx of moderate dehydration (see p. 11)
- Listless/lethargic
- Profuse vomiting or diarrhea
- Significant hypertension:
  - DPB ≥86 if ≤9 years old
  - DPB ≥90 if 10 to 15 years old
  - DPB ≥98 if >15 years old
- Generalized edema
- Hx of congenital urinary disorder
- Hx of renal disease
- Anuria
- Hematuria

Urgent Triage

- Sx of mild dehydration (see p. 11)
- Localized edema of hands, feet, or eyes
- Oliguria
- Persistent vomiting or diarrhea

Nonurgent Triage

- Stable cardiorespiratory and hydration status with:
  * Decreased oral intake
  * Mild reduction in urine output
  * Strong-smelling, concentrated urine
  * Mild vomiting or diarrhea

Interventions

- Complete 1° and 2° survey (see p. 3)
- ✓ GCS (see inside back cover)
- Assess urine for color and amount (diapers per day)

- Obtain urine specimen according to standing orders (see p. 27); if unable to obtain specimen, place urine bag on infants or give specimen cup to older patients

UROLOGIC/RENAL

Protocol **78**   Dysuria

Critical Triage	Acute Triage
• **Any** critical vital sign/parameter (see inside back cover)	• Listless/lethargic • Inconsolable irritability • Fever ≥41° C oral or rectal • Fever ≥38° C rectal in infants ≤10 weeks old • Severe abdominal/flank pain • Inability to void • Frank blood with urination

Urgent Triage

- Hx of renal disease
- Hx of congenital urinary disorder
- Fever ≥38° C to 40.9° C in infants 10 to 12 weeks old
- Moderate abdominal/flank pain
- Noticeable irritability
- Moderate brown or bright red blood mixed with urine
- Considerable difficulty with urination
- Hx of myelomeningocele

Nonurgent Triage

- Stable cardiorespiratory and hydration status with:
  * Fever ≥38° C to 40.9° C in infants >12 weeks old
  * Trace blood in urine
  * Painful urination
- Urination frequency and urgency
- Cloudy urine
- Urine with foul odor
- Toilet-trained child having urinary "accidents"

Interventions

- Complete 1° and 2° survey (see p. 3)
- ✓ GCS (see inside back cover)
- Assess urine for amount, color, odor, and presence of blood
- Percuss flank area to assess for costal vertebral angle (CVA) tenderness

- Obtain routine U/A according to standing orders (see p. 27)
- Administer antipyretics for fever according to standing orders (see pp. 24 and 25)

UROLOGIC/RENAL

Protocol 79 Flank Pain

Critical Triage	**Acute Triage**

Critical Triage

- **Any** critical vital sign/parameter (see inside back cover)
- Agonizing abdominal/flank pain

Acute Triage

- Orthostatic vital signs (see p. 10)
- Severe abdominal/flank pain
- Fever ≥41° C oral or rectal
- Hx of significant abdominal/flank trauma ≤12 hours ago
- Frank blood during urination
- Inability to void

Urgent Triage

- Moderate abdominal/flank pain
- Minor abdominal/flank trauma 12 to 12 hours ago
- Painful urination
- Fever ≥38.3° C to 40.9° C oral or rectal
- Moderate bright red or brown blood mixed with urine
- Hx of renal disease
- Hx of congenital urinary disorder

Nonurgent Triage

- Stable cardiorespiratory and hydration status with:
  * Hx of minor abdominal/flank injury >24 hours ago
  * Increased urinary frequency and urgency
  * Trace blood in urine
  * Cloudy urine

Interventions

- Complete 1° and 2° survey (see p. 3
- Assess urine for color, amount, odor, and presence of blood
- Percuss flank area for CVA tenderness

- Obtain urine specimen according to standing orders (see p. 27)
- Administer antipyretics for fever according to standing orders (see pp. 24 and 25)

UROLOGIC/RENAL

Protocol 80 Hematuria

Critical Triage

- **Any** critical vital sign/parameter (see inside back cover)
- Marked hypertension:
  - * SBP ≥160 if ≤10 years old
    SBP ≥170 if >10 years old

  - * DBP ≥105 if ≤10 years old
    DBP ≥110 if >10 years old

Acute Triage

- Listless/lethargic
- Fever ≥41° C oral or rectal
- Fever ≥38.3° C rectal in infants ≤10 weeks old
- Inconsolable irritability
- Severe abdominal/flank pain
- Frank blood during urination
- Purpura
- Significant hypertension:
  - * DBP ≥86 if ≤9 years old
  - * DPB ≥90 if 10 to 15 years old
  - * DPB ≥98 if >15 years old
- Marked pallor
- Petechial/purpura
- Hx of bleeding disorder
- Hx of congenital urinary disorder
- History of renal disease
- Hx of significant renal or genital trauma ≤12 hours ago

Urgent Triage

- Fever ≥38.3° C to 40.9° C oral or rectal in infants 10 to 12 weeks old
- Moderate abdominal/flank pain
- Noticeable irritability
- Hx of minor renal or genital trauma ≤12 to 24 hours ago
- Urethral foreign body
- Moderate bright red or brown blood mixed with urine

Nonurgent Triage

- Stable cardiorespiratory and neurologic status with:
  * Dysuria
  * Trace blood in urine
  * Increased urinary frequency and urgency
  * Hx of minor renal or genital injury >24 hours ago
- Active menses in puburtal patients

Interventions

- ◆ Complete 1° and 2° survey (see p. 3)
- ◆ ✓ GCS (see inside back cover)
- ◆ Assess urine for amount, color, and presence of blood
- ◆ Assess for difficulty in voiding

- ◆ Assess for Hx of renal or genital trauma
- ◆ Obtain urine specimen according to standing orders (see p. 27)
- ◆ Administer antipyretics for fever according to standing orders (see pp. 24 and 25)

UROLOGIC/RENAL

Protocol **81** Polyuria

Critical Triage

- **Any** critical vital sign/parameter (see inside back cover)
- Kussmaul breathing
- Sx of severe dehydration (see p. 11)
- Stuporous, difficult to arouse

Acute Triage

- Orthostatic vital signs (see p. 10)
- Mild to moderate tachypnea or tachycardia
- Sx of moderate dehydration (see p. 11)
- Listless/lethargic
- Inconsolable irritability
- Hx of recent head trauma
- Severe abdominal pain
- Severe nausea and vomiting
- Dextrose stick 180 to 300 mg/dl
- Hx of diabetes mellitus
- Hx of renal disease

Urgent Triage

- Sx of mild dehydration (see p. 11)
- Excessive thirst
- Noticeable irritability
- Considerable abdominal pain
- Intermittent nausea and vomiting
- Fruity or acetone odor on breath

Nonurgent Triage

- Stable cardiorespiratory and hydration status with:
  * Ingestion of large volume of fluids
  * Increased urinary urgency and frequency
  * Dysuria
  * Minor abdominal pain or stomachache

Interventions

- ◆ Complete 1° and 2° survey (see p. 3)
- ◆ ✓ GCS (see inside back cover)
- ◆ ✓ glucose via finger stick
- ◆ Assess hydration status
- ◆ ✓ urine for glucose or ketones

MUSCULOSKELETAL

Protocol 82   Back Pain

Critical Triage

- **Any** critical vital sign/parameter (see inside back cover)
- Severe respiratory distress (see p. 11)
- Significant back trauma with loss of motor or sensory function
- Hemiparesis of upper or lower extremities
- Cervical spine pain/injury
- Paralysis

Acute Triage

- Fever ≥41° C oral or rectal
- Paresthesia to upper or lower extremities
- Sharp, shooting back pain or pain running down leg
- Significant back trauma ≤12 hours ago
- Significantly decreased ROM in lower extremities
- Inability to bear weight or walk

Urgent Triage

- Minor back trauma ≤12 hours ago
- Moderate back pain
- Ambulates with difficulty

Nonurgent Triage

- Stable cardiorespiratory status with:
  * Minor back injury >12 hours ago
  * Dysuria
  * Minor backache
  * Premenstrual back discomfort

Interventions

- ◆ Complete 1° and 2° survey (see p. 3)
- ◆ ✓ GCS (see inside back cover)
- ◆ Apply cervical collar to patients c/o cervical or spinal pain
- ◆ Assess degree of pain using pain scale (1 to 10)

- ◆ ✓ gross sensory and motor function in extremities
- ◆ Administer antipyretics for fever according to standing orders (see pp. 24 and 25)

MUSCULOSKELETAL

Protocol 83   Cast Problems

Critical Triage

- **Any** critical vital sign/parameter (see inside back cover)
- Neurovascular compromise to affected extremity or limb: ✓ four Ps:
  * Pain out of proportion to injury
  * Pallor
  * Pulselessness
  * Paralysis
- Cyanosis of the affected limb

Acute Triage

- Weak peripheral pulse distal to site of injury
- Cold and mottled skin distal to injury
- Marked swelling distal to injury
- Paresthesia distal to injury
- Absence of feeling distal to injury
- Severe pain of affected limb
- Fever ≥41° C oral or rectal

Urgent Triage

- Moderate pain of affected limb
- Grossly fragmented cast
- Fever 38° C to 40.9° C oral or rectal
- Moderate swelling distal to injury

Nonurgent Triage

- Stable cardiorespiratory and neurovascular status with:
  * Cast discomfort
  * Foul odor from cast
  * Foreign object inside cast
  * Minor crack or break in cast
  * Itching

Interventions

- ◆ Complete 1° and 2° survey (see p. 3)
- ◆ Assess neurovascular status of affected limb
- ◆ Administer antipyretics for fever according to standing orders (see pp. 24 and 25)

- ◆ Splint or sling severely fragmented casts for stability

MUSCULOSKELETAL

Protocol 84 Dislocations

Critical Triage

- **Any** critical vital sign/parameter (see inside back cover)
- Neurovascular compromise to affected extremity or limb; ✓ four Ps:
  * Pain out of proportion to injury
  * Pallor
  * Pulselessness
  * Paralysis
- Multiple traumatic injuries

Acute Triage

- Significantly painful gross dislocation of any joint with decreased ROM
- Musculoskeletal injury to joint or limb with obvious break in skin
- Weak peripheral pulse distal to injury
- Paresthesia distal to injury
- Severe pain in affected limb

Urgent Triage

- Minor musculoskeletal injury to joint or limb ≤12 hours ago with:
  * Minor dislocation of joint
  * Decreased ROM
  * Refusal to bear weight or walk
  * Soft tissue swelling
- Moderate pain in affected limb
- Ecchymosis
- Nursemaid's elbow

Nonurgent Triage

- Stable cardiorespiratory and neurovascular status with minor musculoskeletal injury to joint or limb >12 hours ago

Interventions

- Complete 1° and 2° survey (see p. 3)
- ✓ GCS (see inside back cover)
- ✓ neurovascular status of affected limb
- Use RICE mnemonic:

  R = Rest affected area in comfortable position

  I = Ice application to affected area for 20 to 30 minute intervals; immobilize

  C = Compression: apply elastic bandage to provide support (unless grossly displaced or open fracture) and decrease swelling

  E = Elevate affected limb to decrease swelling
- Refer for radiologic studies according to standing orders (see p. 28)
- Complete trauma score (see Appendix C, p. 324)

MUSCULOSKELETAL

Protocol 85 Fractures

Critical Triage

- **Any** critical vital sign/parameter (see inside back cover)
- Neurovascular compromise of affected extremity or limb: ✓ four Ps:
  * Pain out of proportion to injury
  * Pallor
  * Pulselessness
  * Paralysis
- Multiple traumatic injuries
- Absence of sensation distal to site of injury

Acute Triage

- Obvious dislocation or grossly displaced fracture of limb
- Severe pain, swelling, and decreased ROM of affected limb with decreased peripheral pulse
- Musculoskeletal injury to limb with open break in skin
- Suspected fracture of femur, mandible, pelvis, rib, or scapula
- Paresthesia distal to site of injury
- Marked reduction in sensation distal to injury

Urgent Triage

- Minor musculoskeletal injury to joint or limb ≤12 hours ago with:
  * Decreased ROM
  * Soft tissue swelling
  * Refusal to bear weight
- Moderate pain and swelling of affected limb
- Ecchymosis

Nonurgent Triage

- Stable cardiorespiratory and neurovascular status with minor musculoskeletal injury to joint or limb >12 hours ago

Interventions

- Complete 1° and 2° survey (p. 3)
- ✓ GCS (see inside back cover)
- ✓ neurovascular status of affected limb
- Palpate extremity joint for point tenderness or deformity
- Use RICE mnemonic:

  R = Rest affected area in comfortable position

  I = Ice application to affected area for 20 to 30 minute intervals; immobilize

C = Compression: apply elastic bandage to provide support (unless grossly displaced or open fracture) and decrease swelling

E = Elevate affected limb to decrease swelling

- Keep patient with open Fx of limb NPO
- Refer patient for radiologic studies according to standing orders (see p. 28)
- Complete trauma score (see Appendix C, p. 324)

MUSCULOSKELETAL

Protocol 86 Limping/Refusal to Walk

Critical Triage

- **Any** critical vital sign/parameter (see inside back cover)
- Generalized motor weakness

Acute Triage

- Orthostatic vital signs (see p. 10)
- Significant trauma to hip or limb ≤12 hours ago with:
    * Obvious limb deformity
    * Substantial swelling, severe pain
    * Decreased ROM
- Fever ≥41° C oral or rectal

Urgent Triage

- Minor trauma to hip or limb ≤12 hours ago
- Fever ≥38.3° C oral or rectal
- Refusal to bear weight or walk

Nonurgent Triage

- Stable cardiorespiratory and neurovascular status with:
  * Minor trauma to hip or limb ≥12 hours ago
  * Able to bear weight or walk
  * Afebrile

Interventions

- ◆ Complete 1° and 2° survey (see p. 3)
- ◆ Carefully observe gait while attempting to distract patient with toy
- ◆ Question patient and caretaker for recent Hx of limb or hip trauma

- ◆ If trauma to limb, obtain radiologic studies according to standing orders (see p. 28) after consulting attending MD
- ◆ Administer antipyretics according to standing orders (see pp. 24 and 25)

MUSCULOSKELETAL

Protocol 87 Motor Weakness

Critical Triage

- **Any** critical vital sign/parameter (see inside back cover)
- Stuporous, difficult to arouse
- Generalized motor or sensory weakness
- Hemiparesis
- Severe respiratory distress (see p. 11)
- Slurred speech
- Facial drooping or asymmetry
- Flaccid paralysis
- Absence of sensation
- Hx of head or spinal trauma ≤24 hours ago

Acute Triage

- Sx of moderate dehydration (see p. 11)
- Fever ≥41° C oral or rectal
- Moderate respiratory distress (see p. 11)
- Listless/lethargic
- Focal motor or sensory weakness
- Paresthesia in upper or lower extremities
- Hx of toxic substance ingestion
- Visual impairment
- Ataxia
- Marked reduction in sensation
- Hx of sickle cell disease
- Hx of metabolic disorder
- Hx of head or spinal trauma >24 hours ago

Urgent Triage

- Mild respiratory distress (see p. 11)
- Sx of mild dehydration (see p. 11)
- Sleepy but easily arousable
- Noticeably decreased activity
- Fever ≥38.3° C oral or rectal
- Unequal gross motor strength bilaterally

Nonurgent Triage

- Stable cardiorespiratory and neurovascular status with:
  * Alert, awake, cooperative mental status
  * Normal muscle strength and tone
  * Steady gait

Interventions

- ◆ Complete 1° and 2° survey (see p. 3)
- ◆ ✓ GCS (see inside back cover)
- ◆ ✓ muscle strength and tone
- ◆ ✓ for ingestion of contaminated food or toxic substance
- ◆ Administer antipyretic for fever according to standing orders (see pp. 24 and 25)

MUSCULOSKELETAL

Protocol 88 Strains and Sprains

Critical Triage

- **Any** critical vital sign/parameter (see inside back cover)
- Neurovascular compromise of affected extremity or limb: ✓ four Ps:
  * Pain out of proportion to injury
  * Pallor
  * Pulselessness
  * Paralysis
- Absence of sensation distal to injury

Acute Triage

- Significant trauma to joint or limb ≤12 hours ago
- Significant dislocation or grossly displaced limb or joint
- Severe pain, swelling, and decreased ROM of affected limb or joint
- Decreased peripheral pulse
- Paresthesia distal to injury
- Marked reduction in sensation distal to injury

Urgent Triage

- Minor musculoskeletal injury to joint or limb ≤12 hours ago with:
  * Decreased ROM
  * Refusal to bear weight or walk
  * Soft tissue swelling
  * Moderate pain
  * Ecchymosis
  * Nursemaid's elbow

Nonurgent Triage

- Stable cardiorespiratory and neurovascular status with minor musculoskeletal injury to joint or limb >12 hours ago

Interventions

- ◆ Complete 1° and 2° survey (see p. 3)
- ◆ ✓ neurovascular status of affected limb
- ◆ Use RICE mnemonic:

  R = Rest affected area in comfortable position

  I = Ice application to affected area for 20 to 30 minute intervals; immobilize

  C = Compression: apply elastic bandage to provide support

  (unless grossly displaced or open fracture) and decrease swelling

  E = Elevate affected limb to decrease swelling

- ◆ Keep patient with open Fx of limb NPO
- ◆ Refer for radiologic studies according to standing orders (see p. 28)
- ◆ Complete trauma score (see Appendix C, p. 324)

Critical Triage

Protocol 89
Abrasion

- **Any** critical vital sign/parameter (see inside back cover)
- Stuporous, difficult to arouse
- Petechial/purpuric rash *below* nipple line with fever ≥38.3° C oral or rectal

Acute Triage

- Orthostatic vital signs (see p. 10)
- Fever ≥41° C oral or rectal
- Listless/lethargic
- Marked pallor or ashen color
- Inconsolable irritability
- Fever ≥38.3° C rectal in infants ≤10 weeks old
- Petechial/purpuric rash *below* nipple line with fever <38.3° C oral or rectal
- Severe joint pain, limited ROM, or inability to bear weight, *without* Hx of trauma

Urgent Triage

- Noticeable irritability but consolable
- Localized redness, swelling, warmth, and tenderness surrounding site of injury
- Fever ≥38.3° C to 40.9° C rectal in infants 10 to 12 weeks old
- Copious purulent discharge with pain and swelling
- Red streaks running up extremity proximal to site of injury

Nonurgent Triage

- Stable cardiorespiratory and neurologic status with:
  * Alert, active, cooperative mental status
  * Superficial skin scrape
  * Fever ≥38° C to 40.9° C oral or rectal >12 weeks old

Interventions

- ◆ Complete 1° and 2° survey (see p. 3)
- ◆ ✓ GCS (see inside back cover)
- ◆ Assess injury for signs of cellulitis
- ◆ Administer antipyretics for fever according to standing orders (see pp. 24 and 25)

WOUNDS/TRAUMATIC INJURY

Protocol 90 Avulsion/Amputation

Critical Triage

- **Any** critical vital sign/parameter (see inside back cover)
- Stuporous, difficult to arouse
- Profuse frank bleeding/hemorrhaging
- Hx of bleeding disorder
- Cyanosis distal to injury
- Gross amputation of any digit or limb
- Pulsatile bleeding
- Pulselessness
- Marked pallor
- Paralysis
- Agonizing pain

Acute Triage

- Orthostatic vital signs (see p. 10)
- Severe bleeding
- Gross skin avulsion or degloving
- Weak peripheral pulse distal to injury
- Paresthesia distal to injury
- Dizziness or syncopal episode
- Severe pain

Urgent Triage

- Moderately active bleeding
- Considerable pain
- Full thickness injury to digit or extremity

Nonurgent Triage

- Stable cardiorespiratory status with minor superficial skin abrasion or wound

Interventions

- ◆ Complete 1° and 2° survey (see p. 3)
- ◆ Assess wound for extent of injury, bleeding, exposed muscles or tendons, possible coexisting fractures
- ◆ Apply direct pressure for pulsatile or frank bleeding

- ◆ ✓ pulse distal to injury
- ◆ ✓ GCS (see inside back cover)
- ◆ Bandage wounds with normal saline bulky dressing
- ◆ Preserve amputated or avulsed part by immersing in container of normal sterile saline placed on ice

NOTE: Avulsion, full thickness loss of skin; amputation, traumatic loss of entire digit or limb.

WOUNDS/TRAUMATIC INJURY

Protocol 91 Bites

Critical Triage

- **Any** critical vital sign/parameter (see inside back cover)
- Severe respiratory distress (see p. 11)
- Unusual drooling, dysphagia, or dysphonia
- Inability to speak
- Stuporous, difficult to arouse
- Paralysis
- Profuse frank bleeding/hemorrhaging
- Pulsatile bleeding
- Petechial/purpuric rash with fever ≥38.3° C
- Edema of mouth, lips, or tongue

Acute Triage

- Orthostatic vital signs (see p. 10)
- Moderate respiratory distress (see p. 11)
- Listless/lethargic
- Edema of face or eyes
- Paresthesia
- Dizziness or syncopal episode
- Severe abdominal pain
- Severe nausea or vomiting
- Extensive laceration ≤12 hours ago
- Severe joint pain or swelling
- Fever ≥41° C oral or rectal

Urgent Triage

- Mild respiratory distress (see p. 11)
- Generalized urticarial rash
- Severe puritis
- Moderate nausea or vomiting
- Sizable laceration ≤12 hours ago
- Copious purulent discharge from wound *with* fever ≥38.3° C oral or rectal
- Considerable joint pain or swelling
- Repeat rabies shot prophylaxis

Nonurgent Triage

- Stable cardiorespiratory, neurologic, and hydration status with:
  * Localized redness, swelling, irritation, or itching
  * Fever ≥38.3° C to 40.9° C oral or rectal
  * Localized pain
  * Minor insect, dog, or human bite

Interventions

- Complete 1° and 2° survey (see p. 3)
- ✓ GCS (see inside back cover)
- Assess location size of bite marks
- Assess for systemic reaction
- Assess pain on scale of 1 (none) to 10 (severe)

- Briefly cleanse wound with disinfectant and bandage
- Administer antipyretics for fever according to standing orders (see pp. 24 and 25)

WOUNDS/TRAUMATIC INJURY

Protocol 92   Contusion

Critical Triage

- **Any** critical vital sign/parameter (see inside back cover)
- Severe respiratory distress (see p. 11)
- Head contusion with Hx of bleeding disorder
- Stuporous, difficult to arouse
- Generalized gross motor or sensory weakness
- Absent peripheral pulse

Acute Triage

- Orthostatic vital signs (see p. 10)
- Mild to moderate respiratory distress (see p. 11)
- Listless/lethargic
- Seizure ≤12 hours ago
- Vertigo
- Severe headache
- Severe pain and swelling
- Localized motor or sensory weakness
- Paresthesia distal to injury
- Weak peripheral pulse
- Severe chest or abdominal pain
- Involuntary abdominal guarding with rebound tenderness
- Markedly distended, rigid abdomen
- Persistent vomiting
- Flank pain with hematuria
- Referred shoulder pain
- Marked pallor
- Hx of significant abdominal, chest, extremity, or head trauma ≤12 hours ago
- Hx of bleeding disorder

Urgent Triage

- Moderate chest, abdominal, or flank pain
- Moderate headache
- Hx of minor abdominal, chest, extremity, or head trauma ≤12 hours ago

Nonurgent Triage

- Stable cardiorespiratory and neurologic status with:
  * Minor discomfort, swelling, or bruising of skin
  * Hx of minor abdominal, chest, extremity, or head injury

Interventions

- Complete 1° and 2° survey (see p. 3)
- ✓ GCS (see inside back cover)
- ✓ SpO$_2$
- ✓ pupils
- Assess Hx, mechanism, and extent of blunt injury

- ✓ Hx of bleeding disorders
- Apply ice to affected area for comfort
- ✓ urine for presence of blood
- Complete trauma score (see Appendix C, p. 324)

WOUNDS/TRAUMATIC INJURY

Protocol 93   Gunshot

Critical Triage

- **Any** critical vital sign/parameter (see inside back cover)
- Evidence of *any* respiratory distress (see p. 11)
- Stuporous, difficult to arouse
- Gunshot wound to head, neck, chest, abdomen, or pelvis
- Profuse frank bleeding/hemorrhaging
- Pulsatile bleeding
- Absent or weak peripheral pulse distal to injury
- Paralysis
- Gross motor or sensory weakness
- Paresthesia distal to injury
- Compromised neurovascular status in affected limb
- Clear fluid leak from nose or ear
- Marked pallor
- Agonizing pain

Acute Triage

- Minor BB or low-velocity bullet injury to extremity with stable neurovascular status
- Grazed bullet wound to skin
- Minor active bleeding
- Dizziness or syncopal episode
- Severe pain and swelling
- Reduced sensation to affected limb
- Decreased ROM in affected limb

Urgent Triage

- Old bullet wound with localized redness, pain, or swelling

Nonurgent Triage

- None

Interventions

- ◆ Complete 1° and 2° survey (see p. 3)
- ◆ ✓ GCS (see inside back cover)
- ◆ ✓ SpO$_2$
- ◆ Assess location, size, and mechanism of injury
- ◆ ✓ pulse distal to injury

- ◆ Assess neurovascular status distal to injury
- ◆ Notify appropriate trauma team personnel
- ◆ Complete trauma score (see Appendix C, p. 324)

WOUNDS/TRAUMATIC INJURY

Protocol 94   Hematoma

Critical Triage

- **Any** critical vital sign/parameter (see inside back cover)
- Stuporous, difficult to arouse
- Generalized motor or sensory weakness
- Head trauma with Hx of bleeding disorder
- Petechial/purpuric rash *below* nipple line with fever ≥38.3° C oral or rectal

Acute Triage

- Inconsolable irritability
- Listless/lethargic
- Petechial/purpuric rash *below* nipple line with fever <38.3° C oral or rectal
- Multiple unexplained bruises
- Abnormal bleeding from gums, mouth, nose, or rectum
- Gross hematuria
- Marked pallor
- Localized motor or sensory weakness
- Severe abdominal pain
- Hx of bleeding disorder
- Hx of significant trauma to head, neck, chest, abdomen, pelvis, or extremity ≤12 hours ago

Urgent Triage

- Noticeable irritability but consolable
- Petechial/purpuric rash *above* nipple line
- Moderate abdominal pain
- Moderately painful headache
- C/o "bruising easy" without Hx of trauma
- Hx of minor trauma to head, chest, abdomen, pelvis, or extremity ≤12 hours ago

Nonurgent Triage

- Stable cardiorespiratory and neurologic status with:
  * Localized pain, swelling, or bruising of skin
  * Hx of minor injury to head, chest, abdomen, pelvis, or extremity >12 hours ago

Interventions

- Complete 1° and 2° survey (see p. 3)
- ✓ GCS (see inside back cover)
- Assess lesions for size, color, location, and duration
- Assess if Hx is consistent with mechanism of injury (see p. 7)

- ✓ for Hx of excessive aspirin or nonsteroidal antiinflammatory drug use
- Complete trauma score (see Appendix C, p. 324)

WOUNDS/TRAUMATIC INJURY

Protocol 95 Laceration

Critical Triage

- **Any** critical vital sign/parameter (see inside back cover)
- Profuse frank bleeding/hemorrhaging
- Pulsatile bleeding
- Stuporous, difficult to arouse
- Paralysis
- Absent peripheral pulse distal to injury
- Cyanosis of extremity
- Generalized motor or sensory weakness
- Marked pallor
- Agonizing pain

Acute Triage

- Orthostatic vital signs (see p. 10)
- Severe active bleeding
- Dizziness or syncopal episode
- Localized motor or sensory weakness
- Paresthesia distal to injury
- Weak peripheral pulse distal to injury
- Extensive, traumatic open wound
- Any laceration with open Fx
- Hx of bleeding disorder

Urgent Triage

- Traumatic open wound ≤12 hours old
- Facial wound <24 hours ago
- Moderately active bleeding

Nonurgent Triage

- Stable cardiorespiratory and neurovascular status with:
  * Any open wound >12 hours ago (except facial)
  * Facial wound >24 hours ago
  * Minor superficial abrasion or wound

Interventions

- Complete 1° and 2° survey (see p. 3)
- Apply direct pressure to pulsatile wounds
- ✓ GCS (see inside back cover)
- Assess neurovascular status distal to injury
- ✓ pulse distal to injury

- Assess gross sensory and motor functions
- Inspect wound for foreign body
- Obtain x-ray of injured area for foreign body or concomminant Fx according to standing orders (see p. 28)
- Dress wound with normal saline bulky dressing

WOUNDS/TRAUMATIC INJURY

Protocol 96 Multiple Trauma

Critical Triage

- **Any** critical vital sign/parameter (see inside back cover)
- Severe respiratory distress (see p. 11)
- Frank hemorrhage
- Flail chest response
- Trauma score ≤12
- GCS ≤8 (see inside back cover)
- Stuporous, difficult to arouse
- Hemiparesis/paralysis
- Evidence of spinal cord injury
- High speed crash, 18-inch intrusion on patient side or 24-inch on opposite side of car
- Patient ejected from vehicle
- Vehicle rollover
- Death of same-car occupant
- Patient struck at speed ≥35 mph
- Fall from ≥30 feet or third floor
- Near or complete amputation above or below knee
- Penetrating injury to head, neck, chest, abdomen, or groin, deeper than subcutaneous tissue
- Neurovascular compromise to affected limb

Acute Triage

- Mild to moderate respiratory distress (see p. 11)
- Significant trauma to head, neck, chest, abdomen, or pelvis ≤12 hours ago
- Significant fall of <30 feet
- Gross dislocation or openly displaced fracture of joint or limb
- Seizure ≤12 hours ago
- Listless/lethargic
- Paresthesia
- Minor motor vehicle accident (pedestrian or passenger) with patient c/o cervical neck or back pain
- Focal motor or sensory weakness
- Weak peripherial pulse
- Unexplained injuries in various stages of healing

Urgent Triage

- Minor trauma to head, neck, chest, abdomen, or pelvis ≤12 hours ago
- Obvious dislocation or fracture of joint or limb *without* neurovascular compromise

Nonurgent Triage

- None
- Triage other signs and symptoms

Interventions

- Complete 1° and 2° survey (see p. 3)
- ✓ GCS (see inside back cover)
- ✓ SpO$_2$
- ✓ pupils
- Apply cervical collar for patient c/o cervical spine pain

- Obtain radiologic studies according to standing orders (see p. 28)
- Complete trauma score (see Appendix C, p. 324)

NOTE: If patient has multiple traumatic injuries, immediately transport to resuscitation area for emergency treatment and stabilization.

WOUNDS/TRAUMATIC INJURY

Protocol 97   Puncture/Stab

Critical Triage

- **Any** critical vital sign/parameter (see inside back cover)
- Pulsatile bleeding
- Severe respiratory distress (see p. 11)
- **Any** penetrating injury to chest, abdomen, head, neck, or groin that extends beyond subcutaneous tissue
- Paralysis
- Absent peripheral pulse distal to injury

Acute Triage

- Hx of bleeding disorder
- Localized motor or sensory weakness
- Paresthesia distal to injury
- Weak peripheral pulse distal to injury
- Severe pain, swelling, or bleeding
- Fever ≥41° C oral or rectal

Urgent Triage

- Hx of minor traumatic skin injury ≤12 hours ago
- Moderate pain, swelling, or bleeding
- Copious yellow-green purulent discharge from wound with fever ≥38.3° C oral or rectal

Nonurgent Triage

- Stable cardiorespiratory and neurovascular status with:
  * Hx of minor traumatic skin injury >12 hours ago
  * Minor puncture wound no deeper than epidermal tissue
  * Minor pain, swelling, or bleeding

Interventions

- Complete 1° and 2° survey (see p. 3)
- ✓ GCS (see inside back cover)
- Assess wound for size, depth, location, and extent of injury
- Assess neurovascular status distal to injury
- Inspect wound for foreign body
- Obtain X-ray for wounds with foreign body according to standing orders (see p. 28)
- Bandage wound with normal saline bulky dressing
- Administer antipyretics for fever according to standing orders (see pp. 24 and 25)
- Complete trauma score (see Appendix C, p. 324)

WOUNDS/TRAUMATIC INJURY

Protocol 98   Stings/Envenomations

Critical Triage

- **Any** critical vital sign/parameter (see inside back cover)
- Severe respiratory distress (see p. 11)
- Unusual drooling, dysphagia, or dysphonia
- Inability to speak
- Stuporous, difficult to arouse
- Paralysis
- Generalized motor or sensory weakness
- Edema of mouth, lips, or tongue

Acute Triage

- Orthostatic vital signs (see p. 10)
- Moderate respiratory distress (see p. 11)
- Fever ≥41° C oral or rectal
- Listless/lethargic
- Severe headache
- Paresthesia
- Dizziness or syncopal episode
- Generalized pain with muscle rigidity
- Edema of face or eyes
- Marked pallor
- Severe nausea or vomiting
- Abdominal rigidity
- Severe abdominal pain

Urgent Triage	**Nonurgent Triage**

Urgent Triage

- Mild respiratory distress (see p. 11)
- Generalized urticarial rash
- Severe pruritis
- Moderate nausea or vomiting
- Bite with pustule, edema, and subcutaneous skin discoloration

Nonurgent Triage

- Stable cardiorespiratory and neurologic status with:
  * Localized redness, swelling, or irritation
  * Minor insect bite or sting
  * Localized pain
  * Fever ≥38.3° C to 40.9° C oral or rectal

Interventions

- Complete 1° and 2° survey (see p. 3)
- ✓ GCS (see inside back cover)
- Assess for systemic allergic reaction
- Assess location and size of fang or sting marks
- Assess skin for swelling and color of surrounding tissue
- Assess pain level on scale of 1 (none) to 10 (severe)

- Keep extremity *below* heart if possible
- Remove jewelry or tight fitting clothing from affected extremity
- Keep NPO with severe reactions
- Consult MD for antihistamine for itching
- Administer antipyretics for fever according to standing orders (see pp. 24 and 25)

WOUNDS/TRAUMATIC INJURY

Protocol **99** Suture Removal

Critical Triage	Acute Triage
• None	• None

Urgent Triage

- Unapproximated opened wound with torn or ruptured sutures

Nonurgent Triage

- Stable cardiorespiratory and neurovascular status with:
  * Healing approximated wound with intact sutures
  * Old wound with delayed suture removal

Interventions

- ◆ Complete 1° and 2° survey (see p. 3)
- ◆ Assess integrity of wound
- ◆ Assess wound for signs of infection, redness, swelling, tenderness, discharge, or fever (if infected, see Wound Infection protocol, p. 228)

- ◆ Timetable for suture removal:
  * Eyelids . . . . .3 days
  * Neck . . . . .3 to 4 days
  * Face and scalp . . . . .5 days
  * Trunk and upper extremities . . . . .7 days
  * Lower extremities . .8 to 10 days

WOUNDS/TRAUMATIC INJURY

Protocol 100   Wound Infection (Recheck)

Critical Triage

- **Any** critical vital sign/parameter (see inside back cover)
- Stuporous, difficult to arouse
- Petechial/purpuric rash *below* nipple line with fever ≥38.3° C oral or rectal
- Evisceration
- Gangrene
- Neurovascular compromise in affected limb

Acute Triage

- Orthostatic vital signs (see p. 10)
- Fever ≥41° C oral or rectal
- Listless/lethargic
- Inconsolable irritability
- Fever ≥38° C in infants ≤10 weeks old
- Marked pallor or ashen color
- Petechial/purpuric rash *below* nipple line with fever <38.3° C oral or rectal
- Severe joint pain, limited ROM, or inability to bear weight, *without* Hx of trauma
- Dehiscence

Urgent Triage

- Noticeable irritability but consolable
- Moderate joint pain and swelling
- Considerable redness, edema, warmth, and tenderness of wound area
- Fever ≥38° C to 40.9° C rectal in infants 10 to 12 weeks old
- Copious yellow-green, purulent discharge from wound with fever ≥38.3° C oral or rectal

Nonurgent Triage

- Stable cardiorespiratory and neurologic status with:
  * Minor wound or injury with localized redness, swelling, tenderness, and drainage
  * Any wound, burn, or laceration previously treated and in need of reevaluation or redressing (no signs of infection)

Interventions

- ◆ Complete 1° and 2° survey (see p. 3)
- ◆ ✓ GCS (see inside back cover)
- ◆ Assess wound for signs of infection:
  * Fever
  * Redness
  * Warmth
  * Swelling
  * Drainage
- ◆ Administer antipyretics for fever according to standing orders (see pp. 24 and 25)

DERMATOLOGIC

Protocol **101**   Diaper Rash

Critical Triage	Acute Triage
• **Any** critical vital sign/parameter (see inside back cover)	• Fever ≥41° C oral or rectal • Fever ≥38° C in infants ≤10 weeks old

Urgent Triage

- Fever ≥38° C to 40.9° C in infants 10 to 12 weeks old

Nonurgent Triage

- Stable cardiorespiratory and hydration status with:
  * Fever ≥38° C to 40.9° C in infants >12 weeks old
  * Red, excoriated rash or lesions on groin, genitalia, buttocks, or lower abdomen

Interventions

- ◆ Complete 1° and 2° survey (see p. 3)
- ◆ Administer antipyretics for fever according to standing orders (see pp. 24 and 25)

DERMATOLOGIC

Protocol **102** Measles

Critical Triage

- **Any** critical vital sign/parameter (see inside back cover)
- Severe respiratory distress (see p. 11)
- Stuporous, difficult to arouse
- Sx of severe dehydration (see p. 11)

Acute Triage

- Moderate respiratory distress (see p. 11)
- Fever ≥41° C oral and rectal in any child
- Fever ≥38° C rectal in infants ≤10 weeks old
- Sx of moderate dehydration (see p. 11)
- Listless/lethargic
- Inconsolable irritability
- Severe headache
- Ataxia
- Hx of seizure
- Visual, auditory, or speech disturbances

Urgent Triage

- Mild respiratory distress (see p. 11)
- Fever ≥38° C to 40.9° C rectal in infants 10 to 12 weeks old
- Sx of mild dehydration
- Noticeable irritability but consolable
- Moderately painful headache

Nonurgent Triage

- Stable cardiorespiratory and hydration status with:
  * Maculopapular rash on face or trunk
  * Cough
  * Nasal discharge
  * Conjunctivitis
  * Koplick's spots (white patches) on buccal area
- Fever ≥38° C to 40.9° C rectal or oral in infants >12 weeks old

Interventions

- Complete 1° and 2° survey (see p. 3)
- ✓ GCS (see inside back cover)
- ✓ SpO$_2$
- Assess respiratory and hydration status

- Administer antipyretics for fever according to standing orders (see pp. 24 and 25)

NOTE: If measles are suspected, place patient in respiratory isolation.

DERMATOLOGIC

Protocol **103** Petechiae/Purpura

Critical Triage

- **Any** critical vital sign/parameter (see inside back cover)
- Stuporous, difficult to arouse
- Petechial or purpuric rash *below* nipple line with fever ≥38.3° C oral or rectal
- Profuse frank bleeding/hemorrhaging from any site

Acute Triage

- Orthostatic vital signs (see p. 10)
- Active frank bleeding from nose, mouth, or rectum
- Petechial or purpuric rash *below* nipple line with fever <38.3° C oral or rectal
- Listless/lethargic
- Severe headache
- Hx of seizure
- Nuchal rigidity/stiff neck
- Bulging fontanel
- Marked pallor
- Hematuria
- Hx of oncologic disorder
- Hx of bleeding disorder
- Hx of hematologic disorder

Urgent Triage

- Petechial rash *above* nipple line; afebrile
- Hx of sudden, excessive bruising not related to traumatic injury or active play

Nonurgent Triage

- Stable cardiorespiratory status with:
  * Hx of recent minor trauma with tender, localized eccymotic bruise on skin
  * Bruising easily associated with active play

Interventions

- ◆ Complete 1° and 2° survey (see p. 3)
- ◆ ✓ GCS (see inside back cover)
- ◆ Assess petechial/purpuric rash location (above or below nipple line [above nipple usually associated with crying])†
- ◆ Obtain Hx of purpura lesions; duration, size, and location

- ◆ Question caretaker about use of medications at home: steroids, antibiotics, or aspirin
- ◆ Question caretaker about recent viral illness, immunization, prolonged bleeding after dental extractions, or recent trauma

†Place in respiratory isolation.

DERMATOLOGIC

Protocol **104** Rash with Itching

Critical Triage

- **Any** critical vital sign/parameter (see inside back cover)
- Severe respiratory distress (see p. 11)
- Unusual drooling, dysphagia, or dysphonia
- Sx of severe dehydration (see p. 11)

Acute Triage

- Orthostatic vital signs (see p. 10)
- Moderate respiratory distress (see p. 11)
- Sx of moderate dehydration (see p. 11)
- Inconsolable irritability
- Listless/lethargic
- Edema of face, eyes, tongue, or mouth
- Dizziness or syncopal episode
- Fever ≥41° C oral or rectal
- Fever ≥38° C rectal in infants ≤10 weeks old

Urgent Triage

- Mild respiratory distress (see p. 11)
- Sx of mild dehydration (see p. 11)
- **Any** urticarial, maculopapular, or vesicular rash with Sx of mild dehydration (see p. 11)
- Generalized urticarial rash
- Maculopapular or vesicular rash with severe itching
- Diarrhea or abdominal cramping
- Sx of Kawasaki syndrome: red maculopapular rash with:
  * Unremitting fever
  * Dry, cracked lips
  * Strawberry tongue
  * Swelling or redness of palms of hands and soles of feet
  * Conjunctivitis
  * Joint aches and pain
  * Itching
- Fever ≥38° C to 40.9° C rectal in infants 10 to 12 weeks old

Nonurgent Triage

- Stable cardiorespiratory and hydration status with minor urticarial, vesicular, or maculopapular rash
- Sx of varicella:
  * Red rash with papules, turning into vesicles, which become pustules *with or without* fever†
  * Fever ≥38° C to 40.9° C oral or rectal in children >12 weeks old

Interventions

- ◆ Complete 1° and 2° survey (see p. 11)
- ◆ ✓ GCS (see inside back cover)
- ◆ ✓ for Hx of allergies to foods, medications, or insects

- ◆ Consult MD for order to administer antihistamine as needed
- ◆ Administer antipyretics for fever according to standing orders (see pp. 24 and 25)

---

†Isolate any patient with Sx of varicella

DERMATOLOGIC

Protocol 105   Rash without Itching

Critical Triage

- **Any** critical vital sign/parameter (see inside back cover)
- Severe respiratory distress (see p. 11)
- Sx of severe dehydration (see p. 11)
- Unusual drooling, dysphagia, or dysphonia
- Petechial or purpuric rash *below* nipple line with fever ≥38.3° C oral or rectal

Acute Triage

- Moderate respiratory distress (see p. 11)
- Sx of moderate dehydration (see p. 11)
- Listless/lethargic
- Petechial or purpuric rash *below* nipple line *without* fever <38.3° C or Hx of trauma†
- Maculopapular/petechial hemorrhagic rash *with* fever ≥38.3° C and vomiting, malaise, myalgia, intense headache
- Fever ≥41° C oral or rectal
- Fever ≥38° C to 40.9° C rectal in infants ≤10 weeks old

Urgent Triage

- Mild respiratory distress (see p. 11)
- Sx of mild dehydration (see p. 11)
- Petechial or purpuric rash *above* nipple line *without* fever[†]
- Fever ≥38° C to 40.9° C rectal in infants 10 to 12 weeks old
- Sx of measles: Maculopapular rash on face and then trunk with:
  * Fever
  * Cough
  * Coryza (copious nasal discharge)
  * Conjunctivitis
  * Koplik's spots (white patches on buccal area)

Nonurgent Triage

- Stable cardiorespiratory and hydration status with:
  * Minor vesicular or maculopapular rash
- Fever ≥38° C to 40.9° C oral or rectal in children >12 weeks old

Interventions

- ◆ Complete 1° and 2° survey (see p. 3)
- ◆ ✓ GCS (see inside back cover)
- ◆ Inspect skin and buccal mucosa for rash or lesions

- ◆ ✓ for Hx of allergic reaction to foods, medications, or insects
- ◆ Administer antipyretics for fever according to standing orders (see pp. 24 and 25)

[†]Examine skin and isolate any patient with petechial rash or Sx of measles.

DERMATOLOGIC

Protocol 106   Urticaria (Hives)

Critical Triage	Acute Triage

Critical Triage

- **Any** critical vital sign/parameter (see inside back cover)
- Severe respiratory distress (see p. 11)
- Unusual drooling, dysphagia, or dysphonia
- Inability to speak

Acute Triage

- Fever ≥41° C oral or rectal
- Moderate respiratory distress (see p. 11)
- Profuse nausea and vomiting
- Severe abdominal pain
- Urticarial rash with swelling of face, lips, eyes, or tongue
- Severe headache
- Fever ≥38° C rectal in infants ≤10 weeks old
- Inconsolable irritability

Urgent Triage

- Generalized urticarial rash with severe itching
- Mild respiratory distress (see p. 11)
- Moderate nausea and vomiting
- Abdominal cramping
- Fever 38° C to 40.9° C rectal in infants 10 to 12 weeks old
- Irritable but consolable

Nonurgent Triage

- Stable cardiorespiratory and hydration status with:
  * Localized urticarial rash
  * Insect bite
  * Minor itching
  * Fever 38° C to 40.9° C oral or rectal in children >12 weeks old

Interventions

- Complete 1° and 2° survey (see p. 3)
- ✓ GCS (see inside back cover)
- ✓ SpO$_2$
- Inspect skin and mouth for edema, lesions, and rash

- Consult MD for antihistamine order
- Administer antipyretics for fever according to standing orders (see pp. 24 and 25)

DERMATOLOGIC

Protocol **107**   Varicella

Critical Triage	Acute Triage

Critical Triage

- **Any** critical vital sign/parameter (see inside back cover)
- Sx of severe dehydration (see p. 11)
- Stuporous, difficult to arouse

Acute Triage

- Fever ≥41° C oral or rectal
- Orthostatic vital signs (see p. 10)
- Sx of moderate dehydration (see p. 11)
- Fever ≥38° C rectal in infants ≤10 weeks old
- Listless/lethargic
- Unconsolable irritability
- Nuchal rigidity/stiff neck
- Bulging anterior fontanel
- Intense headache
- Hx of seizure
- Visual, auditory, or speech disturbance

Urgent Triage

- Sx of mild dehydration (see p. 11)
- Fever ≥38° C to 40.9° C rectal in infants 10 to 12 weeks old
- Noticeable irritability but consolable
- Painful headache
- Severe itching
- Open, extremely infected lesions with pain and swelling

Nonurgent Triage

- Stable cardiorespiratory and hydration status with:
  * Vesicular lesions becoming pustular
  * Mild to moderate itching
  * Fever ≥38° C to 40.9° C oral or rectal in children >12 weeks old

Interventions

- ◆ Complete 1° and 2° survey (see p. 3)
- ◆ Assess hydration status
- ◆ ✓ GCS (see inside back cover)
- ◆ Administer antipyretics for fever according to standing orders (see pp. 24 and 25)

NOTE: If varicella is suspected, place patient in respiratory isolation.

HEMATOLOGIC/ONCOLOGIC

Protocol 108 Acquired Bleeding Disorders (DIC, HSP, ITP)

Critical Triage

- **Any** critical vital sign/parameter (see inside back cover)
- Stuporous, difficult to arouse
- Petechial or purpuric rash *below* nipple line with fever ≥38.3° C oral or rectal
- Agonizing headache
- Generalized motor or sensory weakness
- Hx of idiopathic thrombocytopenic purpura (ITP) with head trauma

Acute Triage

- Orthostatic vital signs (see p. 10)
- Listless/lethargic
- Inconsolable irritability
- Fever ≥41° C oral or rectal
- Petechial or purpuric rash *below* nipple line with fever <38.3° C oral or rectal
- Sudden onset of marked pallor or jaundice
- Localized motor or sensory weakness
- Weak peripheral pulse
- Severe headache
- Hematuria
- Hx of ITP with active bleeding

Urgent Triage

- Petechial/purpuric rash *above* nipple line with or without fever ≥38.3° C to 40.9° C oral or rectal
- Moderately painful headache
- Noticeable irritability
- Sudden onset of noticeable pallor or jaundice
- Hx of ITP with minimal bleeding

Nonurgent Triage

- Stable cardiorespiratory and neurologic status with:
  * Awake, alert, cooperative mental status
  * Hx of ITP with bleeding at home

Interventions

- Complete 1° and 2° survey (see p. 3)
- ✓ GCS (see inside back cover)
- Obtain Hx of lesions: duration, size, location, or blanching
- ✓ mucous membranes and conjunctiva for pallor

- Question caretaker about recent bacterial or viral illness and immunizations
- Administer antipyretics for fever according to standing orders (see pp. 24 and 25)

HEMATOLOGIC/ONCLOGIC

Protocol 109 — Inherited Bleeding Disorders (Hemophilia, von Willebrand Disease)

Critical Triage

- **Any** critical vital sign/parameter (see inside back cover)
- Hx of head trauma ≤24 hours ago
- Profuse, frank bleeding
- Pulsatile bleeding
- Marked pallor

Acute Triage

- Hx of head trauma >24 hours ago
- Soft tissue trauma with obvious bleeding hematoma, contusion, or laceration
- Painful swelling of joint with decreased ROM
- Active rectal bleeding
- Active oral bleeding
- Hematuria
- Marked pallor
- Epistaxis
- Hemoptysis

Urgent Triage

- Reported Hx of bleeding from mouth, gums, or rectum

Nonurgent Triage

- None
- Triage other Sx

Interventions

- ◆ Complete 1° and 2° survey (see p. 3)
- ◆ ✓ GCS (see inside back cover)
- ◆ For profuse bleeding, apply pressure dressing and elevate extremity

- ◆ Bandage open wounds with NSS bulky dressing
- ◆ Splint soft tissue injury in comfortable position and elevate extremity if possible

HEMATOLOGIC/ONCOLOGIC

Protocol **110** Jaundice

Critical Triage

- **Any** critical vital sign/parameter (see inside back cover)
- Stuporous, difficult to arouse
- Petechial/purpuric rash *below* nipple line with fever ≥38.3° C oral or rectal
- Sx of severe dehydration (see p. 11)

Acute Triage

- Severe jaundice
- Orthostatic vital signs (see p. 10)
- Sx of moderate dehydration (see p. 11)
- Listless/lethargic
- Inconsolable irritability
- Fever ≥41° C oral or rectal
- Fever ≥38° C rectal in infants ≤10 weeks old
- Cool, mottled extremities
- Marked pallor
- Petechial or purpuric rash *below* nipple line with fever <38.3° C oral or rectal
- Seizure ≤12 hours ago
- Severe abdominal pain
- Painful, distended abdomen
- Profuse vomiting

Urgent Triage

- Moderate jaundice
- Sx of mild dehydration (see p. 11)
- Seizure >12 hours ago
- Fever ≥38° C to 40.9° C rectal in infants 10 to 12 weeks old
- Noticeable irritability
- Persistent vomiting
- Newborn/infant ≤8 weeks old with jaundice
- Hx of hemolytic disease
- Hx of liver disease
- Hx of sickle cell disease

Nonurgent Triage

- Stable cardiorespiratory and hydration status with:
  * Fever ≥38° C to 40.9° C oral or rectal in children >12 weeks old
- Dysuria
- Intermittent vomiting
- Mild jaundice

Interventions

- ◆ Complete 1° and 2° survey (see p. 3)
- ◆ ✓ GCS (see inside back cover)
- ◆ Assess degree of jaundice in skin, sceera, mucous membranes, and darkening of urine

- ◆ Administer antipyretics for fever according to standing orders (see pp. 24 and 25)

HEMATOLOGIC/ONCOLOGIC

Protocol 111 Oncologic Disorders

Critical Triage

- **Any** critical vital sign/parameter (see inside back cover)
- Severe respiratory distress (see p. 11)
- Petechial rash *with* fever ≥38.3° C oral or axillary[†]
- Stuporous, difficult to arouse
- Cool, mottled extremities
- Weak peripheral pulses

Acute Triage

- Orthostatic vital signs (see p. 10)
- Fever ≥38.3° C oral or axillary
- Listless/lethargic
- Petechial rash *without* fever[†]
- Moderate respiratory distress (see p. 11)
- Sx of moderate dehydration (see p. 11)
- Hx of neutropenia[†]
- Marked pallor or anemia
- Immunocompromised
- Severe headache
- Persistent vomiting or diarrhea

Urgent Triage

- Mild respiratory distress (see p. 11)
- Sx of mild dehydration (see p. 11)
- Reliable Hx of fever at home

Nonurgent Triage

- None
- Triage other Sx

Interventions

- ◆ Complete 1° and 2° survey (see p. 3)
- ◆ ✓ GCS (see inside back cover)
- ◆ ✓ SpO_2
- ◆ ✓ for petechial rash on trunk and extremities

- ◆ ✓ for recent blood counts (e.g., absolute neutrophil count (ANC) <1000)
- ◆ Administer antipyretic for fever according to standing orders (see p. 24)

---

†Place in respiratory isolation.

HEMATOLOGIC/ONCOLOGIC

Protocol **112** Pallor/Anemia

Critical Triage

- **Any** critical vital sign/parameter (see inside back cover)
- Severe respiratory distress (see p. 11)
- Marked pallor of mucous membranes
- Petechial or purpuric rash *below* nipple line with fever ≥38.3° C oral or rectal

Acute Triage

- Orthostatic vital signs (see p. 10)
- Significant pallor of mucous membranes
- Listless/lethargic
- Painful, distended abdomen
- Hematuria
- Inconsolable irritability
- Severe jaundice
- Generalized bruising not associated with trauma
- Petechial or purpuric rash *below* nipple line with fever <38.3° C oral or rectal†
- Pallor of mucous membranes
- Cool, mottled extremities
- Weak peripheral pulses

Urgent Triage

- Noticeable pallor of nail beds and conjunctiva
- Failure to thrive; poor feeding and poor weight gain
- Noticeable irritability but consolable
- Localized bruising not associated with trauma
- Somnolence

Nonurgent Triage

- Stable cardiorespiratory and neurologic status with:
  * Pink mucous membranes
  * Alert, awake, and cooperative mental status
  * Consolable
  * Generalized malaise

Interventions

- ◆ Complete 1° and 2° survey (see p. 3)
- ◆ ✓ GCS (see inside back cover)
- ◆ Examine skin and mucous membranes for pallor or jaundice

- ◆ ✓ for Hx of glucose-6-phosphate dehydrogenase deficiency (G_6PD)
- ◆ ✓ SpO_2

---

†Isolate any patient with petechial or purpuric rash.

HEMATOLOGIC/ONCOLOGIC

Protocol 113 Sickle Cell Anemia

Critical Triage

- **Any** critical vital sign/parameter (see inside back cover)
- Severe respiratory distress (see p. 11)
- Slurred speech
- Generalized or focal motor or sensory weakness
- Facial drooping or asymmetry
- Debilitating headache
- Hemiparesis

Acute Triage

- Orthostatic vital signs (see p. 10)
- Fever ≥38.3° C oral or rectal
- Moderate respiratory distress (see p. 11)
- Vasoocclusive crisis pain
- Priapism
- Severe headache
- Marked pallor
- Listless/lethargic
- Intense left upper quadrant pain with involuntary guarding

Urgent Triage

- Low-grade fever (38° C to 38.2° C oral or rectal)
- Mild, localized crisis discomfort *without* swelling; able to use affected extremity

Nonurgent Triage

- Stable cardiorespiratory and neurologic status with awake, alert, cooperative mental status
- Triage other Sx

Interventions

- Complete 1° and 2° survey (see p. 3)
- ✓ GCS (see inside back cover)
- ✓ SpO$_2$
- Ask patient to rate crisis pain on scale of 1 (none) to 10 (severe)

- Administer antipyretics for fever according to standing orders (see pp. 24 and 25)

IMMUNOLOGIC

Protocol **114** Allergic Reaction

Critical Triage	Acute Triage
• **Any** critical vital sign/parameter (see inside back cover)	• Moderate respiratory distress (see p. 11)
• Severe respiratory distress (see p. 11)	• Edema of face or eyes
• Unusual drooling, dysphagia, or dysphonia	• Wheezing
• Inability to speak	• Dizziness or syncopal episode
• Irregular heartbeat	• Severe abdominal pain
• Edema of mouth, lips, or tongue	• Profuse nausea and vomiting

Urgent Triage

- Mild respiratory distress (see p. 11)
- Generalized urticarial rash
- Severe pruritis (itching)
- Persistent nausea and vomiting
- Abdominal cramping

Nonurgent Triage

- Stable cardiorespiratory status with:
  - * Localized urticarial rash
  - * Mild pruritis (itching)
  - * Insect bites with localized response

Interventions

- ◆ Complete 1° and 2° survey (see p. 3)
- ◆ ✓ SpO$_2$
- ◆ Inspect skin and mouth for edema, lesions, and rash
- ◆ Call local Poison Control Center (#_____-_____)
- ◆ Consult MD for order to administer antihistamine as needed

IMMUNOLOGIC

Protocol 115   Special Immunology (HIV)

Critical Triage

- **Any** critical vital sign/parameter (see inside back cover)
- Stuporous, difficult to arouse
- Petechial or purpuric rash *below* nipple line with fever ≥38.3° C oral or rectal
- Severe respiratory distress (see p. 11)
- Sx of severe dehydration (see p. 11)
- Cold, mottled extremities
- Weak peripheral pulse

Acute Triage

- Orthostatic vital signs (see p. 10)
- Moderate respiratory distress (see p. 11)
- Sx of moderate dehydration (see p. 11)
- Profuse vomiting or diarrhea
- Fever ≥38° C oral or rectal
- Listless/lethargic
- Inconsolable irritability
- Petechial/purpuric rash *below* nipple line with fever <38.3° C

Urgent Triage

- Noticeable irritability
- Mild respiratory distress (see p. 11)
- Sx of mild dehydration (see p. 11)
- Chronic failure to thrive
- Intermittent vomiting or diarrhea

Nonurgent Triage

- None
- Triage other Sx

Interventions

- ◆ Complete 1° and 2° survey (see p. 3)
- ◆ ✓ GCS (see inside back cover)
- ◆ ✓ SpO$_2$
- ◆ Administer antipyretics for fever according to standing orders (see pp. 24 and 25)

- ◆ Document *special immunology* on triage form instead of *AIDS* or *HIV* to maintain patient confidentiality

INFECTIOUS DISEASE

Protocol 116 Fever in Infants ≤10 Weeks Old

Critical Triage

- **Any** critical vital sign/parameter (see inside back cover)
- Severe respiratory distress (see p. 11)
- Sx of severe dehydration (see p. 11)
- Petechial or purpuric rash *below* nipple line *with* fever ≥38° C rectal†
- Stuporous, difficult to arouse

Acute Triage

- Fever ≥38° C rectal in infants ≤10 weeks old
- Moderate respiratory distress (see p. 11)
- Sx of moderate dehydration (see p. 11)
- Petechial or purpuric rash *below* nipple line *with* fever <38° C rectal†
- Sx of moderate dehydration (see p. 11)
- Nuchal rigidity/stiff neck†
- Bulging anterior fontanel
- Inconsolable irritability
- Hx of seizure ≤12 hours ago
- Listless/lethargic
- Dextrose stick 40 to 80 mg/dl

Urgent Triage

- Mild respiratory distress (see p. 11)
- Noticeable irritability but consolable
- Reliable Hx of fever ≥38° C rectal at home
- Sx of mild dehydration (see p. 11)
- Hx seizure >12 hours ago

Nonurgent Triage

- Stable cardiorespiratory and hydration status with alert, awake, consolable mental status

Interventions

- ◆ Complete 1° and 2° survey (see p. 3)
- ◆ ✓ GCS (see inside back cover)
- ◆ ✓ SpO$_2$
- ◆ ✓ glucose via finger stick
- ◆ Administer antipyretic for fever

according to standing orders (see pp. 24 and 25)

- ◆ Undress patient to one layer of loose clothing
- ◆ Offer Pedialyte or formula to patient if *not* vomiting

---

†Examine skin for petechial rash and place patient in respiratory isolation.

INFECTIOUS DISEASE

Protocol **117**   Fever in Patients >10 Weeks Old

Critical Triage

- **Any** critical vital sign/parameter (see inside back cover)
- Severe respiratory distress (see p. 11)
- Stuporous, difficult to arouse
- Petechial/purpuric rash *below* nipple line *with* fever ≥38.3° C oral or rectal*
- Sx of severe dehydration (see p. 11)

Acute Triage

- Moderate respiratory distress (see p. 11)
- Sx of moderate dehydration (see p. 11)
- Fever ≥41° C oral or rectal
- Petechial/purpuric rash *below* nipple line with temperature <38.3° C oral or rectal†
- Nuchal rigidity/stiff neck†
- Bulging anterior fontanel
- Inconsolable irritability
- Listless/lethargic
- Hx of neutropenia (ANC <1000)
- Hx of oncologic disorder and fever ≥38.3° C
- Hx of seizure ≤12 hours ago
- Hx of sickle cell disease and fever ≥38.3° C oral or rectal
- Hx of ventroperitoneal shunt and fever ≥38.3° C

Urgent Triage

- Fever ≥38° C rectal in infants 10 to 12 weeks old
- Mild respiratory distress (see p. 11)
- Sx of mild dehydration (see p. 11)
- Hx of seizure >12 hours ago
- Hx of sickle cell disease; temperature <38.3° C oral or rectal
- Noticeable irritability but consolable

Nonurgent Triage

- Stable cardiorespiratory and hydration status with fever ≥38° C to 40.9° C oral or rectal in children >12 weeks old

Interventions

- Complete 1° and 2° survey (see p. 3)
- ✓ GCS (see inside back cover)
- ✓ SpO$_2$
- Undress patient to one layer of loose clothes

- Administer antipyretic for fever according to standing orders (see pp. 24 and 25)
- Offer Pedialyte, formula, or juice to patient if *not* vomiting

---

†Examine skin for petechial rash and place in respiratory isolation.

INFECTIOUS DISEASE

Protocol 118 Positive Blood Culture

Critical Triage

- **Any** critical vital sign/parameter (see inside back cover)
- Severe respiratory distress (see p. 11)
- Stuporous, difficult to arouse
- Petechial or purpuric rash *below* nipple line with fever ≥38.3° C oral or rectal
- Cold, mottled extremities
- Weak peripheral pulse

Acute Triage

- Orthostatic vital signs (see p. 10)
- Mild to moderate respiratory distress (see p. 11)
- Listless/lethargic
- Fever ≥38° C oral or rectal in any child
- Petechial or purpuric rash *below* nipple line with fever <38.3° C oral or rectal
- Inconsolable irritability
- Stiff neck/nuchal rigidity†
- Bulging anterior fontanel
- High-pitched cry

Urgent Triage

- Low grade fever ≤38° C oral or rectal in any child
- Noticeable irritability
- Petechial or purpuric rash *above* nipple line; afebrile

Nonurgent Triage

- None
- Triage other Sx

Interventions

- ◆ Complete 1° and 2° survey (see p. 3)
- ◆ ✓ SpO_2
- ◆ ✓ GCS (see inside back cover)
- ◆ ✓ for petechial or purpuric rash
- ◆ Administer antipyretics for fever according to standing orders (see pp. 24 and 25)

---

†Place in respiratory isolation.

METABOLIC/ENDOCRINE

Protocol **119** Diabetes

Critical Triage

- **Any** critical vital sign/parameter (see inside back cover)
- Kussmaul's sign for irregular breathing
- Stuporous, difficult to arouse
- Severe respiratory distress (see p. 11)
- Sx of severe dehydration (see p. 11)
- Cold, mottled extremities
- Weak peripheral pulse
- Dextrose stick <40 mg/dl or >300 mg/dl and symptomatic

Acute Triage

- Orthostatic vital signs (see p. 10)
- Moderate respiratory distress (see p. 11)
- Sx of moderate dehydration (see p. 11)
- Listless/lethargic
- Profuse vomiting
- Large amount of ketones or glucose in urine
- Dextrose stick 180 to 300 mg/dl, or 40 to 80 mg/dl and symptomatic
- Significant abdominal pain
- Inconsolable irritability
- Marked weight loss
- Ataxia
- Vertigo
- Visual disturbances

Urgent Triage

- Mild respiratory distress (see p. 11)
- Sx of mild dehydration (see p. 11)
- Intermittent vomiting
- C/o "poorly controlled sugar at home" with dextrose stick 120 to 179 mg/dl
- Malaise
- Sudden weight loss
- Polydipsia or polyphagia
- Glucosuria
- Somnolence

Nonurgent Triage

- None
- Triage other Sx

Interventions

- Complete 1° and 2° survey (see p. 3)
- ✓ GCS (see inside back cover)
- Assess respiratory status for Kussmaul's sign
- ✓ glucose via finger stick

- ✓ for ketones on breath and in urine

METABOLIC/ENDOCRINE

Protocol 120 Hypoglycemia

Critical Triage

- **Any** critical vital sign/parameter (see inside back cover)
- Stuporous, difficult to arouse
- Severe respiratory distress (see p. 11)
- Sx of severe dehydration (see p. 11)

Acute Triage

- Orthostatic vital signs (see p. 10)
- Moderate respiratory distress (see p. 11)
- Sx of moderate dehydration (see p. 11)
- Inconsolable irritability
- Seizure <12 hours ago
- Severe headache
- Severe hunger, tremors, or sweating
- Dextrose stick 40 to 80 mg/dl
- Hx of diabetes
- Hx of metabolic disorder

Urgent Triage

- Mild respiratory distress (see p. 11)
- Sx of mild dehydration (see p. 11)
- Malaise
- Seizure >12 hours ago
- Moderate headache
- Moderate hunger, tremors, or sweating
- Noticeable irritability but consolable

Nonurgent Triage

- Stable cardiorespiratory and neurologic status with:
  * Awake, alert, cooperative mental status
  * Mild headache
  * Increased hunger or thirst

Interventions

- ◆ Complete 1° and 2° survey (see p. 3)
- ◆ ✓ GCS (see inside back cover)
- ◆ ✓ glucose via finger stick
- ◆ ✓ urine for ketones
- ◆ Administer juice or fluids if gag reflex is intact

METABOLIC/ENDOCRINE

Protocol **121** Metabolic Disorder

Critical Triage

- **Any** critical vital sign/parameter (see inside back cover)
- Stuporous, difficult to arouse
- Severe respiratory distress (see p. 11)
- Sx of severe dehydration (see p. 11)
- Cold, mottled extremities
- Weak peripheral pulse
- Dextrose stick <40 mg/dl, or >300 mg/dl and symptomatic

Acute Triage

- Orthostatic vital signs (see p. 10)
- Moderate respiratory distress (see p. 11)
- Sx of moderate dehydration (see p. 11)
- Listless/lethargic
- Profuse vomiting
- Significant abdominal pain
- Seizure ≤12 hours ago
- Inconsolable irritability
- Ataxia
- Dextrose stick 40 to 80 mg/dl and symptomatic
- Fever >41° C oral or rectal
- Fever ≥38° C in infants ≤10 weeks old
- Fever in patient with central line in place
- Central line dysfunction

Urgent Triage

- Mild respiratory distress (see p. 11)
- Sx of mild dehydration (see p. 11)
- Intermittent vomiting
- Malaise
- Seizure >12 hours ago
- Chronic failure to thrive
- Noticeable irritability
- Gross motor delay
- Fever >38° C to 40.9° C in infants >10 weeks old

Nonurgent Triage

- None
- Triage other Sx

Interventions

- ◆ Complete 1° and 2° survey (see p. 3)
- ◆ ✓ GCS (see inside back cover)
- ◆ ✓ SpO$_2$
- ◆ ✓ glucose via finger stick

- ◆ ✓ for Hx of food intolerance
- ◆ ✓ for odorous breath or urine
- ◆ Administer antipyretics for fever according to standing orders (see pp. 24 and 25)

TOXICOLOGIC

Protocol 122 Alcohol Ingestion

Critical Triage	Acute Triage

Critical Triage

- **Any** critical vital sign/parameter (see inside back cover)
- Stuporous, difficult to arouse
- Severe respiratory distress (see p. 11)
- Marked tachycardia or bradypnea
- Seizure ≤1 hour ago
- Dextrose stick <40 mg/dl
- Combative, uncontrollable behavior
- Gross motor or sensory impairment

Acute Triage

- Mild to moderate tachycardia
- Mild to moderate bradypnea or tachypnea
- Hx of alcohol ingestion ≤24 hours ago
- Profuse nausea and vomiting
- Listless/lethargic
- Seizure ≤24 hours ago
- Staggering gait
- Ataxia
- Slurred speech
- Uncoordinated gross motor function
- Delirium or disorientation
- Dextrose stick 40 to 80 mg/dl

Urgent Triage

- Hx of alcohol ingestion 24 to 48 hours ago
- Mild headache
- Mild nausea and vomiting
- Stomachache

Nonurgent Triage

- Stable cardiorespiratory and neurologic status with:
  * Hx of alcohol ingestion >48 hours ago
  * Awake, alert, cooperative mental status
  * No other Sx

Interventions

- Complete 1° and 2° survey (see p. 3)
- ✓ GCS (see inside back cover)
- ✓ pupils
- ✓ glucose via finger stick
- ✓ gag reflex
- ✓ motor function
- ✓ time of ingestion
- Call local poison control center (#_____-_____)
- See Appendix G (p. 328) for toxicologic reference information

TOXICOLOGIC

Protocol **123**   Carbon Monoxide Poisoning

Critical Triage	Acute Triage

Critical Triage

- **Any** critical vital sign/parameter (see inside back cover)
- Severe respiratory distress (see p. 11)
- Marked dyspnea, tachypnea, tachycardia, or hypotension
- Irregular heartbeat
- Stuporous, difficult to arouse
- Generalized motor or sensory weakness
- Singed nasal hairs or soot around nares or mouth
- House-fire victim

Acute Triage

- Mild to moderate respiratory distress (see p. 11)
- Mild to moderate tachypnea, tachycardia, or hypotension
- Carbon monoxide exposure ≤24 hours ago
- Severe headache
- Listless/lethargic
- Delirium or disorientation
- Extreme nausea and vomiting
- Seizure ≤24 hours ago
- Noticeable irritability
- Ataxia
- Dizziness
- Cherry red skin color
- Hx of syncopal episode

Urgent Triage

- Carbon monoxide exposure 24 to 48 hours ago with:
  * Mild headache
  * Cranky but consolable mental status
- Seizure >24 hours ago

Nonurgent Triage

- Stable cardiorespiratory and neurologic status with:
  * Carbon monoxide exposure >48 hours ago
  * Awake, alert, cooperative mental status
  * No other Sx

Interventions

- Complete 1° and 2° survey (see p. 3)
- ✓ GCS (see inside back cover)
- ✓ pupils
- ✓ time of exposure
- Call local poison control center (#_____-_____)

- ✓ for Hx of house fire or faulty furnace
- See Appendix G (p. 328) for toxicologic reference information

NOTE: Pulse oximetry to check hemoglobin saturation may be normal and cannot be used as an accurate measure of oxygenation.

TOXICOLOGIC

Protocol **124** Drug Ingestion

Critical Triage

- **Any** critical vital sign/parameter (see inside back cover)
- Stuporous, difficult to arouse
- Severe respiratory distress (see p. 11)
- Irregular heartbeat
- Crushing chest pain
- Combative, uncontrollable behavior
- Gross motor or sensory impairment

Acute Triage

- Mild to moderate respiratory distress (see p. 11)
- Mild to moderate tachycardia or bradycardia
- Mild to moderate hypertension or hypotension
- Hx of drug ingestion ≤24 hours ago
- Listless/lethargic
- Delirium or disorientation
- Seizure ≤24 hours ago
- Ataxia
- Staggering gait
- Pupil changes (dilated or pinpoint)
- Inconsolable irritability
- Torticollis
- Tongue protrusion or heaviness
- Paresthesia
- Chest pain
- Visual impairment
- Tremors
- Heart palpitations
- Profuse nausea and vomiting
- Syncopal episode

Urgent Triage

- Hx of ingestion 24 to 48 hours ago with:
  * Headache
  * Mild nausea and vomiting
- Seizure >24 hours ago

Nonurgent Triage

- Stable cardiorespiratory and neurologic status with:
  * Drug ingestion >48 hours ago
  * Awake, alert, cooperative mental status
  * No other Sx

Interventions

- Complete 1° and 2° survey (see p. 3)
- ✓ GCS (see inside back cover)
- ✓ SpO$_2$
- ✓ pupils
- ✓ gag reflex

- ✓ Hx for class of drug ingested
- ✓ time of ingestion
- Call local poison control center (#_____-_____)
- See Appendix G (p. 328) for toxicologic reference information

TOXICOLOGIC

Protocol 125 Inhalation Injury

Critical Triage

- **Any** critical vital sign/parameter (see inside back cover)
- Stuporous, difficult to arouse
- Severe respiratory distress (see p. 11)
- Crushing chest pain
- Irregular heartbeat
- Unusual drooling, dysphagia, or dysphonia
- Combative, uncontrollable behavior

Acute Triage

- Mild to moderate respiratory distress (see p. 11)
- Mild to moderate tachycardia or bradycardia
- Mild to moderate hypertension or hypotension
- Hx of toxic inhalation ≤24 hours ago
- Severe chest pain
- Heart palpitations
- Severe headache
- Ataxia
- Listless/lethargic
- Visual impairment
- Delirium or disorientation
- Seizure ≤24 hours ago
- Syncopal episode

Urgent Triage

- Hx of toxic inhalation 24 to 48 hours ago with:
  - * Mild headache
  - * Mild nausea or vomiting
- Seizure >24 hours ago

Nonurgent Triage

- Stable cardiorespiratory and neurologic status with:
  - * Hx of toxic inhalation >48 hours ago
  - * Awake, alert, cooperative mental status
  - * No other Sx

Interventions

- ◆ Complete 1° and 2° survey (see p. 3)
- ◆ ✓ SpO$_2$
- ◆ ✓ GCS (see inside back cover)
- ◆ ✓ pupils
- ◆ ✓ Hx for type of inhaled substance
- ◆ ✓ time of exposure

- ◆ Call local poison control center (#_____-_____)
- ◆ See Appendix G (p. 328) for toxicologic reference information

TOXICOLOGIC

Protocol 126 Toxic Substance Ingestion

Critical Triage	Acute Triage
• **Any** critical vital sign/parameter (see inside back cover)	• Mild to moderate respiratory distress (see p. 11)
• Stuporous, difficult to arouse	• Mild to moderate tachycardia or bradycardia
• Severe respiratory distress (see p. 11)	• Mild to moderate hypertension or hypotension
• Unusual drooling, dysphagia, or dysphonia	• Hx of toxic substance ingestion ≤24 hours ago
• Marked changes in visual acuity	• Seizure ≤24 hours ago
• Paralysis or hemiparesis	• Listless/lethargic
• Gross motor or sensory impairment	• Severe headache
• Combative, uncontrollable behavior	• Ataxia
	• Staggering gait
	• Paresthesia
	• Delirium or disorientation
	• Persistent choking, coughing, or gagging
	• Severe abdominal pain
	• Profuse nausea and vomiting
	• Blurred or double vision
	• Burns or blisters of mouth and oral mucosa
	• Tremors

Urgent Triage

- Hx of toxic substance ingestion 24 to 48 hours ago with:
  - * Mild headache
  - * General malaise
  - * Mild nausea or vomiting
- Seizure >24 hours ago

Nonurgent Triage

- Stable cardiorespiratory and neurologic status with:
  - * Hx of toxic substance ingestion >48 hours ago
  - * Awake, alert, cooperative mental status
  - * No other Sx

Interventions

- ◆ Complete 1° and 2° survey (see p. 3)
- ◆ ✓ GCS (see inside back cover)
- ◆ ✓ SpO$_2$
- ◆ ✓ pupils
- ◆ ✓ time of ingestion
- ◆ Call local poison control center (#_____-_____)

- ◆ Do **not** induce vomiting
- ◆ ✓ for toxic odor on breath or clothes
- ◆ ✓ for burns of mouth and oral mucosa
- ◆ See Appendix G (p. 328) for toxicologic reference information

THERMAL

Protocol 127 Chemical Burn

Critical Triage

- **Any** critical vital sign/parameter (see inside back cover)
- Chemical substance in eye
- Severe respiratory distress (see p. 11)
- Unusual drooling, dysphagia, or dysphonia
- Major burn:
  * Partial thickness >20% total body surface area (TBSA)
  * Partial thickness >10% TBSA

Acute Triage

- Mild to moderate respiratory distress (see p. 11)
- Moderate burn:
  * Partial thickness 10% to 20% TBSA
  * Full thickness 3% to 10% TBSA
- Extensive burns to face, ears, hands, feet, or perineum
- Burns to mouth, lip, tongue, or mucosa

Urgent Triage

- Minor burn:
  * Superficial-partial thickness <10% TBSA
  * Full thickness <3% TBSA
- Minor superficial burns to mouth, lip, tongue, or mucosa *without* respiratory distress

Nonurgent Triage

- Stable cardiorespiratory and neurovascular status with:
  * Minor localized burn >24 hours old
  * Minor, localized, superficial (first degree) burn

Interventions

- Complete 1° and 2° survey (see p. 3)
- ✓ SpO$_2$
- ✓ GCS (see inside back cover)
- Remove all patient's clothing and jewelry
- Rinse wound with copious amounts of normal saline and apply normal saline bulky dressing

- Calculate depth and severity of burn using charts (see p. 16)
- Ask patient to rate pain on scale of 1 (none) to 10 (severe)
- Obtain Hx from patient or rescue to identify chemical agent
- Health care providers should wear protective gear during process of chemical decontamination

NOTE: Extent of burn may be difficult to determine initially and may worsen.

THERMAL

Protocol 128 Electrical Burn

Critical Triage

- **Any** critical vital sign/parameter (see inside back cover)
- Hx of cardiorespiratory arrest at scene
- Severe respiratory distress (see p. 11)
- Stuporous, difficult to arouse
- Irregular heartbeat
- Crushing chest pain
- Major burn:
  * Partial thickness >20% TBSA
  * Full thickness >10% TBSA
- Neurovascular compromise to affected limb
- Hemiparesis or paralysis
- Gross motor or sensory weakness
- High-voltage injury
- Lightning injury

Acute Triage

- Mild to moderate respiratory distress (see p. 11)
- Moderate burn:
  * Partial thickness 10% to 20% TBSA
  * Full thickness 3% to 10% TBSA
- Extensive burns to face, ears, hands, feet, or perineum
- Burns to mouth, lip, tongue, or mucosa
- C/o heart palpitations
- Hx of loss of consciousness
- Disorientation
- Seizure ≤12 hours ago
- Paresthesia
- Localized motor or sensory weakness
- Gross bone deformity or dislocation

Urgent Triage

- Minor burn:
  * Superficial-partial thickness <10% TBSA
  * Full thickness <3% TBSA
- Minor superficial burns to mouth, lip, tongue, or mucosa *without* respiratory distress

Nonurgent Triage

- Stable cardiorespiratory and neurovascular status with:
  * Minor localized burn >24 hours old
  * Minor, localized, superficial (first degree) burn

Interventions

- ◆ Complete 1° and 2° survey (see p. 3)
- ◆ ✓ GCS (see inside back cover)
- ◆ ✓ for evidence of burn entrance or exit wounds
- ◆ Assess neurovascular status of affected limb
- ◆ Elevate affected limb to reduce edema
- ◆ Inquire about voltage of current and duration of contact with electricity

- ◆ ✓ for possible coexisting fractures and obtain radiologic studies according to standing orders (p. 28)
- ◆ Calculate depth and severity of burn using chart (see p. 16)
- ◆ Bandage wound with normal saline bulky dressing
- ◆ Test urine for blood to assess for myoglobinuria

NOTE: Electrical injuries may appear superficial but have extensive underlying tissue damage.

THERMAL

Protocol 129 Smoke Inhalation

Critical Triage

- **Any** critical vital sign/parameter (see inside back cover)
- Hx of cardiorespiratory arrest at scene
- Severe respiratory distress (see p. 11)
- Coughing up carbonaceous sputum
- Marked dyspnea
- Stuporous, difficult to arouse
- Singed nasal hairs or soot around nares or mouth
- Major burn:
  * Partial thickness >20% TBSA
  * Full thickness >10% TBSA
- Unusual drooling, dysphagia, or dysphonia
- Generalized motor or sensory weakness

Acute Triage

- Mild to moderate respiratory distress (see p. 11)
- Mild to moderate tachypnea or tachycardia
- Moderate burn:
  * Partial thickness 10% to 20% TBSA
  * Full thickness 3% to 10% TBSA
- Extensive burns to face, ears, hands, feet, or perineum
- Severe headache
- Listless/lethargic
- Delirium/disorientation
- Noticeable irritability
- Ataxia
- Cherry red skin color

Urgent Triage

- Painful headache
- Cranky but consolable
- Dizziness
- Minor burn:
  * Superficial-partial thickness <10% TBSA
  * Full thickness <3% TBSA

Nonurgent Triage

- Stable cardiorespiratory and neurovascular status with:
  * Minor localized burn >24 hours old
  * Minor localized superficial (first degree) burn

Interventions

- ◆ Complete 1° and 2° survey (see p. 3)
- ◆ Administer 100% oxygen
- ◆ ✓ GCS (see inside back cover)
- ◆ ✓ time of exposure
- ◆ Remove patient's clothing and jewelry

- ◆ Calculate depth and severity of burn using charts (see p. 16)
- ◆ Bandage wound with normal saline bulky dressing

NOTE: Pulse oximetry to check hemoglobin saturation may be normal and cannot be used as an accurate measure of oxygenation.

THERMAL

Protocol **130** Thermal Burn

Critical Triage

- **Any** critical vital sign/parameter (see inside back cover)
- Severe respiratory distress (see p. 11)
- Major burn:
  * Partial thickness >20% TBSA
  * Full thickness >10% TBSA
- Unusual drooling, dysphagia, or dysphonia
- Singed nasal hairs or soot around nares or mouth
- Hx of being in house fire
- Marked dyspnea

Acute Triage

- Mild to moderate respiratory distress (see p. 11)
- Moderate burn:
  * Partial thickness 10% to 20% TBSA
  * Full thickness 3% to 10% TBSA
- Extensive burns to face, ears, hands, feet, or perineum
- Burns to mouth, lip, tongue, or mucosa

Urgent Triage

- Minor burn:
  * Superficial-partial thickness <10% TBSA
  * Full thickness <3% TBSA
- Minor superficial burns to mouth, lip, tongue, or mucosa *without* respiratory distress

Nonurgent Triage

- Stable cardiorespiratory and neurovascular status with:
  * Minor localized burn >24 hours old
  * Minor localized superficial (first degree) burn

Interventions

- Complete 1° and 2° survey (see p. 3)
- ✓ GCS (see inside back cover)
- Remove patient's clothing and jewelry
- Calculate depth and severity of burn using chart (see p. 16)
- Rinse wound with normal saline and apply normal saline bulky bandage
- Ask patient to rate pain on scale of 1 (none) to 10 (severe)

NOTE: Pulse oximetry to check hemoglobin saturation may be normal and cannot be used as an accurate measure of oxygenation.

ENVIRONMENTAL

Protocol **131**   Frost Bite

Critical Triage	Acute Triage

Critical Triage

- **Any** critical vital sign/parameter (see inside back cover)
- Stuporous, difficult to arouse
- Severe respiratory distress (see p. 11)
- Neurovascular compromise of affected area or limb: ✓ four Ps:
  * Pallor
  * Pulselessness
  * Paralysis
  * Pain out of proportion to injury
- Cold, hard, cyanotic skin without sensation

Acute Triage

- Weak peripheral pulse distal to injury
- Cold, white skin with waxy appearance
- Paresthesia
- Reduced sensation
- Severe pain and swelling
- Severe burning

Urgent Triage

- Localized cool, pale discoloration of skin with sensation
- Moderate pain
- Moderate burning
- Minor localized tingling or numbness

Nonurgent Triage

- Stable cardiorespiratory and neurovascular status with:
  * Localized itching
  * Minor skin discomfort, redness, or swelling with sensation

Interventions

- ◆ Complete 1° and 2° survey (see p. 3)
- ◆ ✓ GCS (see inside back cover)
- ◆ ✓ neurovascular status of affected area or limb
- ◆ ✓ duration of exposure to cold

- ◆ Elevate extremity in comfortable position
- ◆ Do *not* rub affected area (handle area gently)

ENVIRONMENTAL

Protocol **132**   Heat Illness

Critical Triage

- **Any** critical vital sign/parameter (see inside back cover)
- Stuporous, difficult to arouse
- Sx of severe dehydration (see p. 11)
- Fever ≥41° C oral or rectal and Hx of prolonged exposure in hot environment
- Marked confusion or agitation
- Hemiparesis

Acute Triage

- Orthostatic vital signs (see p. 10)
- Sx of moderate dehydration (see p. 11)
- Delirium or disorientation
- Listless/lethargic
- Severe headache
- Profuse nausea and vomiting
- Paresthesia
- Uncoordinated gross motor function
- Fever ≥38.3° C oral or rectal and Hx of prolonged exposure in hot environment
- Generalized weakness
- Severe muscle cramps
- Seizure ≤12 hours ago
- Inconsolable irritability

Urgent Triage

- Sx of mild dehydration (see p. 11)
- Extreme thirst
- Intermittent muscle cramps
- Moderately painful headache
- Seizure >12 hours ago
- Noticeable irritability but consolable
- Intermittent nausea and vomiting

Nonurgent Triage

- Stable cardiorespiratory, neurologic, and hydration status with:
  * Mild thirst
  * Malaise
  * Sweaty, moist skin
  * Localized muscle cramps

Interventions

- Complete 1° and 2° survey (see p. 3)
- ✓ GCS (see inside back cover)
- Monitor temperature closely
- Remove constrictive clothing

- Keep patient in cool, quiet environment
- For conscious, nonvomiting patients, offer electrolyte-balanced oral solution (Pedialyte or Gatorade)

ENVIRONMENTAL

Protocol 133 Hypothermia

Critical Triage

- **Any** critical vital sign/parameter (see inside back cover)
- Stuporous, difficult to arouse
- Temperature ≤35° C rectal
- Slow, irregular heartbeat
- Marked respiratory depression
- Sluggish, dilated pupils
- Marked pallor
- Cold, mottled extremities
- Weak peripheral pulse

Acute Triage

- Temperature 35° C to 36° C oral or rectal
- Neonate <4 weeks old with subnormal temperature
- Marked fatigue
- Generalized motor or sensory weakness
- Uncoordinated gross motor function
- Cool, pale, mottled skin
- Listless/lethargic
- Delirium or disorientation

Urgent Triage

- Temperature 36° C to 36.4° C rectal
- Malaise
- Noticeable irritability but consolable
- Chilly with considerable shivering

Nonurgent Triage

- Stable cardiorespiratory and neurologic status with:
  * Normothermia
  * Awake, alert, cooperative mental status

Interventions

- ◆ Complete 1° and 2° survey (see p. 3)
- ◆ ✓ GCS (see inside back cover)
- ◆ ✓ Hx for duration of exposure to cold
- ◆ ✓ if patient recently had anything

  cold to drink by mouth
- ◆ If oral temperature is subnormal, recheck rectally
- ◆ Remove wet clothing
- ◆ Wrap in warm blankets and place patient in warm environment

NOTE: When obtaining oral temperature, make sure patient has had nothing cold to drink at least 15 minutes before assessment.

ENVIRONMENTAL

Protocol 134   Radiation Injury[†]

Critical Triage

- **Any** critical vital sign/parameter (see inside back cover)
- Severe respiratory distress (see p. 11)
- Marked hypotension
- Frank bleeding/hemorrhage
- Stuporous, difficult to arouse
- Generalized motor or sensory weakness
- Petechial or purpuric rash
- Extensive radiation burn to skin (erythema, ulceration, gangrenous appearance)

Acute Triage

- Orthostatic vital signs (see p. 10)
- Mild to moderate respiratory distress (see p. 11)
- Severe bleeding
- Listless/lethargic
- Ataxia
- Seizure ≤12 hours ago
- Nausea, vomiting, or diarrhea
- Generalized fatigue
- Localized radiation burn to skin (erythema, ulceration, gangrenous appearance)

	Urgent Triage		Nonurgent Triage

Urgent Triage

- None

Nonurgent Triage

- None

Interventions

- ◆ Complete 1° and 2° survey (see p. 3)
- ◆ ✓ GCS (see inside back cover)
- ◆ ✓ Hx for type of radiation and duration of exposure
- ◆ Radiation precautions

†Immediately place in isolation with special radioactive precautions.

PSYCHOLOGIC

Protocol **135** Behavior Changes

Critical Triage

- **Any** critical vital sign/parameter (see inside back cover)
- Stuporous, difficult to arouse
- Combative, uncontrollable behavior†

Acute Triage

- Delirium/disorientation
- Confused, unable to follow commands
- Seizure <12 hours ago
- Hostile or aggressive behavior†
- Patient in police custody†
- Hx of head trauma
- Hx of toxic substance ingestion
- Hx of seizure disorder
- Hx of ventriculoperitoneal shunt

Urgent Triage

- Seizure >12 hours ago
- Sudden onset of behavioral changes
- Agitated behavior or suicidal ideation[†]
- Medical clearance for psychiatric admission
- Hx of psychiatric disorder

Nonurgent Triage

- Stable cardiorespiratory and neurologic status with awake, alert, cooperative mental status

Interventions

- ◆ Complete 1° and 2° survey (see p. 3)
- ◆ ✓ GCS (see inside back cover)
- ◆ ✓ pupils
- ◆ See Psychosocial Interviewing Techniques (p. 6)

[†]All hostile, aggressive patients in police custody or with suicidal ideation need one-to-one supervision

PSYCHOLOGIC

Protocol 136 Psychosocial Disorder

Critical Triage

- **Any** critical vital sign/parameter (see inside back cover)
- Stuporous, difficult to arouse
- Combative, uncontrollable behavior

Acute Triage

- Clear intent to harm self or plan and lethal means with intent to die (see intervention 1.0)
- Failed suicide attempt before arrival (see intervention 1.1)
- Active hallucinations, delusions, disorganized thinking, marked disorientation, aggressive or destructive behavior (see intervention 1.2)

Urgent Triage

- Self-destructive thoughts but no plan, intent, or means (see intervention 2.0)

- Decreased ability to focus, agitation, slight disorientation (see intervention 2.1)

Nonurgent Triage

- Stable cardiorespiratory and neurologic status with alert, awake, cooperative mental status

Interventions

- ◆ Complete 1° and 2° survey (see p. 3)
- ◆ ✓ GCS (see inside back cover)
- ◆ Complete psychosocial interview (see p. 6)
- ◆ (1.0 and 1.1) Accompany patient to room close to nurses' station and place on 1:1 supervision with ED staff; remove sharp or dangerous objects from environment
- ◆ (1.2) Notify security; accompany patient to room and use safety

restraints as needed, with 1:1 supervision

- ◆ (2.0) Accompany patient to room close to nursing station and place on 1:1 supervision with family member
- ◆ (2.1) Place patient in area of decreased stimulation; use clear, calm directions; make behavioral contracts with patient

SOCIAL

Protocol 137 Abandoned Child

Critical Triage

- **Any** critical vital sign/parameter (see inside back cover)
- Stuporous, difficult to arouse
- Sx of severe dehydration (see p. 11)
- Severe cachexia (malnourished)

Acute Triage

- Orthostatic vital signs (see p. 10)
- Sx of moderate dehydration (see p. 11)
- Listless/lethargic
- Significant muscle wasting and malnutrition

Urgent Triage

- Sx of mild dehydration (see p. 11)
- Hx of abandonment

Nonurgent Triage

- None
- Triage other Sx

Interventions

- ◆ Complete 1° and 2° survey (see p. 3)
- ◆ ✓ GCS (see inside back cover)
- ◆ Notify hospital social services department and charge nurse of patient's status

SOCIAL

Protocol 138 Physical Abuse/Neglect

Critical Triage

- **Any** critical vital sign/parameter (see inside back cover)
- Stuporous, difficult to arouse
- Severe respiratory distress (see p. 11)
- Sx of severe dehydration (see p. 11)
- Multiple traumatic injuries
- Severe burns to face, trunk, and extremities >15% TBSA
- Fracture with neurovascular compromise

Acute Triage

- Moderate respiratory distress (see p. 11)
- Sx of moderate dehydration (see p. 11)
- Significant head trauma ≤12 hours ago
- Listless/lethargic
- Unexplainable large surface burns to face, trunk, extremities, or perineum 10% to 15% TBSA
- Multiple unexplained bruises, contusions, or lacerations
- Seizure ≤12 hours ago
- Displaced, open fracture or obvious femur fracture
- Bilious vomiting
- Battle's sign (ecchymosis behind ear)
- Raccoon eyes (periorbital ecchymosis)

Urgent Triage

- Mild respiratory distress (see p. 11)
- Sx of mild dehydration (see p. 11)
- Minor head trauma ≤24 hours ago *without* neurologic compromise
- Abandoned child
- Localized minor burns to face, trunk, extremities, or perineum <10% TBSA
- Localized unexplained bruises, contusions, lacerations, or fractures
- Seizure >12 hours ago
- Hematuria

Nonurgent Triage

- None

Interventions

- Complete 1° and 2° survey (see p. 3)
- ✓ GCS (see inside back cover)
- Splint and dress all fractures, burns, or open wounds
- Carefully document caretaker's explanation of injuries
- Document on triage form "R/O SCAN" (rule out suspected child abuse and neglect) to preserve patient confidentiality

- Document percent of burns using Lund/Browder chart (see p. 6)
- Inform hospital social worker, charge nurse, and attending MD of patient's condition
- Refer to SCAN interviewing techniques (see p. 6)
- Complete trauma score (see Appendix C, p. 324)

SOCIAL

Protocol 139 Sexual Abuse

Critical Triage

- **Any** critical vital sign/parameter (see inside back cover)
- Multiple traumatic injuries

Acute Triage

- Lethargic/listless
- Seizure ≤12 hours ago
- Head trauma ≤12 hours ago
- Unexplained frank vaginal bleeding
- Vaginal laceration
- Frank rectal bleeding
- Rectal laceration

Urgent Triage

- C/o sexual assault occurring ≤72 hours ago in children <12 years old
- Genital bruising, swelling, or irritation
- Rectal pain or fissure
- Unexplained sexually transmitted disease (STD)
- Unexplained vaginal or urethral discharge or lesions
- Caretaker concern about possible sex assault

Nonurgent Triage

- Stable cardiorespiratory status with sexual assault occurred >72 hours ago to child <12 years old

Interventions

- ◆ Complete 1° and 2° survey (see p. 3)
- ◆ ✓ GCS (see inside back cover)
- ◆ Refer to SCAN interview techniques (see p. 6) to obtain Hx
- ◆ Examine skin for unexplained bruising, swelling, or lesions
- ◆ Carefully document patient's explanation of chief complaint

- ◆ Document on triage form "R/O CODE R" (rule out suspected sexual abuse) to preserve patient confidentially
- ◆ Notify hospital social worker, charge nurse, and attending MD of patient's condition as needed

NOTE: Children ≥12 years old who are stable and c/o sexual assault should be referred to adult facility for care (#_____-_____) (see p.6).

GENERAL

Protocol **140**   Care of the Adult Patient

Critical Triage

- Cyanosis
- Apnea
- Unstable vital signs
- Severe respiratory distress (see p. 11)
- Stuporous, difficult to arouse
- Gross motor or sensory weakness
- Cold, mottled extremities
- Weak peripheral pulse
- Crushing chest pain
- Debilitating headache
- Marked hypertension
- Dextrose stick <40 or >300 mg/dl
- **Any** life- or limb-threatening illness or injury

Acute Triage

- Orthostatic vital signs (see p. 10)
- Moderate respiratory distress (see p. 11)
- Syncopal episode
- Seizure <12 hours ago
- **Any** significant health problem that could potentially become life or limb threatening

Urgent Triage

- Mild respiratory distress (see p. 11)
- **Any** health problem not potentially life or limb threatening

Nonurgent Triage

- Awake, alert, cooperative mental status
- **Any** minor health problem with stable cardiorespiratory and neurologic status

Interventions

- ◆ Complete 1° and 2° survey (see p. 3)
- ◆ ✓ GCS (see inside back cover)
  - Critical: Immediately treat and stabilize patient before transferring to adult facility
  - Acute: Evaluate and treat before transferring to adult facility

- Urgent and Nonurgent: Consult attending MD and refer patient to adult facility

NOTE: The transferring facility must comply with COBRA regulations before patient transfer or referral to another facility.

GENERAL

Protocol 141 Central Line Dysfunction (Broviac, Infusaport, PIC Line)

Critical Triage

- **Any** critical vital sign/parameter (see inside back cover)
- Severe respiratory distress (see p. 11)
- Petechial or purpuric rash *below* nipple line with fever ≥38.3° C oral or rectal†
- Irregular heartbeat
- Pleuritic chest pain radiating to shoulders
- Weak peripheral pulse
- Cold, mottled extremities
- Dextrose stick <40 mg/dl or >300 mg/dl

Acute Triage

- Orthostatic vital signs (see p. 10)
- Fever ≥38.3° C oral or rectal
- Moderate respiratory distress (see p. 11)
- Petechial or purpuric rash *below* nipple line with fever <38.3° C oral or rectal†
- Listless/lethargic
- Inconsolable irritability
- Muffled or distant heart sounds
- Hemoptysis
- Dextrose stick 40 to 80 mg/dl
- Hx of metabolic disorder

Urgent Triage

- Noticeable irritability but consolable
- Low grade fever (38° C to 38.2° C) oral or rectal
- Localized infection at catheter site
- Catheter fluid leak
- Difficulty obtaining central line access
- Unable to flush catheter
- Broken central line catheter
- Hx of gastrointestinal disorder
- Hx of immunocompromise
- Hx of oncologic disorder†
- Hx of sickle cell disease

Nonurgent Triage

- None
- Triage other Sx

Interventions

- ◆ Complete 1° and 2° survey (see p. 3)
- ◆ ✓ GCS (see inside back cover)
- ◆ ✓ for petechial rash
- ◆ ✓ glucose via finger stick

- ◆ Administer antipyretics for fever according to standing orderls (see pp. 24 and 25)
- ◆ ✓ security of central line dressing; clamp tubing

---

†Place in respiratory isolation.

GENERAL

Protocol **142** Ill Appearing Infant

Critical Triage

- **Any** critical vital sign/parameter (see inside back cover)
- Severe respiratory distress (see p. 11)
- Sx of severe dehydration (see p. 11)
- Stuporous, difficult to arouse
- Petechial or purpuric rash *below* nipple line with fever ≥38.3° C rectal
- Irregular heartbeat
- Hypothermia
- Marked pallor

Acute Triage

- Moderate respiratory distress (see p. 11)
- Sx of moderate dehydration (see p. 11)
- Fever ≥38° C in infants ≤10 weeks old
- Fever ≥41° C oral or rectal
- Marked pallor or jaundice
- Unconsolable irritability
- Listless/lethargic
- Distended, rigid abdomen
- Vomiting coffee ground or bilious fluids
- Bloody diarrhea or "currant jelly" stool
- Cool extremities/weak peripheral pulses
- Head trauma <12 hours ago
- Nuchal rigidity/stiff neck†
- Bulging anterior fontanel
- Petechial or purpuric rash *below* nipple line with fever <38.3° C rectal†
- Generalized edema
- Seizure ≤12 hours ago
- Dextrose stick 40 to 80 mg/dl

Urgent Triage

- Fever ≥38° C rectal in infants 10 to 12 weeks old
- Mild respiratory distress (see p. 11)
- Sx of mild dehydration (see p. 11)
- Minor head trauma >12 hours ago
- Failure to thrive; poor feeding and weight gain
- Seizure >12 hours ago
- Noticeable irritability but consolable
- Profuse vomiting
- Petechial or purpuric rash *above* nipple line *without* fever
- Unexplained bruising without reliable Hx of trauma

Nonurgent Triage

- Stable cardiorespiratory and hydration status with:
  * Awake, alert, consolable mental status
  * Intermittent vomiting or diarrhea
  * Fever ≥38° C to 40.9° C oral or rectal in children >12 weeks old

Interventions

- Complete 1° and 2° survey (see p. 3)
- ✓ GCS (see inside back cover)
- ✓ SpO$_2$

- ✓ glucose via finger stick
- Administer antipyretics for fever according to standing orders (see pp. 24 and 25)

†Examine skin for petechial or purpuric rash and place in respiratory isolation.

Section V

Appendices

APPENDIX A

Job Description for the Primary Triage Nurse

General Responsibilities

The primary triage nurse is directly responsible to the nurse manager, attending physician, and charge nurse of the ED. Responsibilities include but are not limited to the following:

- Initiates and completes the nursing process
- Assesses, analyzes, plans, intervenes, and evaluates the quality of care delivered to all incoming patients to the triage area
- Complies with established triage policies and procedures for the delivery of safe and effective triage care
- Maintains awareness of all incoming patients to the triage area
- Prioritizes patients in need of immediate triage care and determines those patients whose triage evaluation may be delayed
- Completes a primary and secondary survey on all patients in triage as necessitated by their condition (see p. 3).
- Initiates the triage documentation record (see Appendix C) and maintains patient confidentiality
- Collects vital signs, subjective, and objective triage information including allergies, medication, and immunization status
- Administers appropriate triage protocols including diagnostic studies (X-ray studies, etc.)
- Administers standing triage medications
- Administers appropriate first aid measures

(e.g., splinting, applying ice, dressing wounds).
- Assigns the patient a triage category (Critical, Acute, Urgent, or Nonurgent) based upon the child's severity of illness in accordance with established triage protocols.

Professional Qualifications

- Licensed as a professional nurse in the state in which she/he practices
- Knowledge of basic life support techniques
- Knowledge of pediatric advanced life support or advanced cardiac life support techniques preferred
- Certified emergency nurse preferred
- Satisfactory completion of a triage instructional program
- Satisfactory completion of a preceptor triage training program and on-going evaluation
- Minimum 6 months ED experience

Personal Qualifications

- Exercises rapid critical thinking skills in formulating triage assessments
- Demonstrates excellent prioritization skills
- Maintains composure and is able to adapt to stressful and rapidly changing environments
- Utilizes interpersonal skills to effectively communicate with patients, families, health care providers, and community

Specific Responsibilities

- Collaborates with the charge nurse and attending physician to facilitate the triage process
- Provides ongoing reevaluation and assessments for triaged patients waiting for further ED evaluation
- Provides patients and families with a caring, reassuring attitude and assists them with questions, concerns, or patient issues

APPENDIX B

Triage Competency Behaviors

Directions: Please check the appropriate box that applies to the given behavior. Add additional comments as necessary in the space provided.

Critical Competency Behaviors	Date	S*	D*	Comments
Completed triage course				
Minimum 16 hour triage precepting time				
Triage posttest				
15 chart self-audit				
Consistently demonstrates the following behaviors:				
Documents appropriate subjective data relevant to the patients' complaint				
Documents appropriate objective data that supports the designated triage priority				
Accurately documents primary and secondary survey				
Documents normal and abnormal vital signs and parameters				

*S, Satisfactory; D, deficient

continued

Triage Competency Behaviors—Continued

Critical Competency Behaviors	Date	S*	D*	Comments
Documents supporting triage information: Patient Name				
Age				
Allergies				
Past medical/surgical history				
Medications/last dose				
Exposure to communicable disease				
Means of arrival: rescue, car				
Documents arrival and triage times				
Demonstrates effective communication skills: Utilizes principals of therapeutic communication				
Introduces self				
Maintains eye contact with the patient and family				
Informs patients and families in a caring, reassuring manner of: waiting time				
patient's assessed condition				
opportunity for patients and families to return to the triage desk if the patient's condition worsens while waiting				

Critical Competency Behaviors	Date	S*	D*	Comments
Demonstrates the ability to use interdepartmental communication devices in triage, including:				
Intercom				
Panic button				
Telephone				
Security				
Collects rescue run sheets from rescue/EMS personnel and places with patient chart				
Demonstrates an ability to assess and prioritize patients to be triaged and reevaluates patients awaiting further treatment				
Implements appropriate triage interventions:				
Antipyretics (acetaminophen or ibuprofen)				
X-ray studies				
Pulse oximetry				
Cervical collars				
Urine collection				
Wound care				
Ice and splinting				
First aid				
Isolates patients with suspected communicable diseases (e.g., varicella, measles, TB, pertussis) and notifies charge nurse or nurse covering that zone				
Isolates patients in reverse flow rooms who are				

continued

Triage Competency Behaviors—Continued

CRITICAL COMPETENCY BEHAVIORS	DATE	S*	D*	COMMENTS
immunosuppressed (e.g., patients with cancer, AIDS, or who have had a recent transplant) and notifies charge nurse or nurse covering that zone				
Identifies suspected abuse cases, demonstrates knowledge of the physical and psychologic signs of abuse and notifies social work in a timely way Child abuse (R/O SCAN)				
Sexual abuse (R/O Code R)				
Demonstrates knowledgeable and accurate physical assessment skills, data gathering, and documentation skills with various patient complaints: Age appropriate vital signs				
Respiratory assessment				
breath sounds				
pulse oximetry				
skin color				
Cardiac assessment				
quality of pulses				
capillary refill				
quality of skin (dry, clammy)				
Level of consciousness				
pupillary assessment				
sensory and motor function				

CRITICAL COMPETENCY BEHAVIORS	DATE	S*	D*	COMMENTS
Hydration status				
mucus membranes				
Bowel sounds				
Wound assessment				
Demonstrates sound working knowledge of triage classification system				
Critical				
Acute				
Urgent				
Nonurgent				
Fast track				
Knowledgeable of trauma alert criteria				
Demonstrates ability to make appropriate referrals:				
Diagnostic studies (Lab, X-ray)				
Outpatient				
Pediatric ambulatory clinics				
Fast track				
Demonstrates understanding of "red flag" triage findings:				
Alterations in airway				
Breathing and circulation				
Loss of consciousness				
Fever in infant ≤10 weeks old				
Acute visual changes				
Weak, frail, crying				
Petechiae/purpura				

continued

Triage Competency Behaviors—Continued

CRITICAL COMPETENCY BEHAVIORS	DATE	S*	D*	COMMENTS
Pulse oximetry <93%				
Acute testicular pain				
Meningeal signs (nuchal rigidity)				
Abnormal vital signs				
Listless/lethargic				
Provides comfort measures when appropriate:				
Formula/diapers				
Pedialyte, juice				
Blankets or sheets				
Makes appropriate contact with support services:				
Social worker				
Security				
Police				
Poison control				
Demonstrates knowledge of cultural diversity in health care practices of patients & families				
Incorporates patient teaching when appropriate				
Demonstrates ability to adjust triage pace, volume dependent				
Demonstrates legible handwriting				
Seeks assistance from charge nurse when necessary				

Critical Competency Behaviors	Date	S*	D*	Comments
Consults with ED attending physician when necessary:				
Unknown rashes				
Uncertain trauma decision				
Uncertain about X-ray results				
AMA				
Interacts with security when appropriate:				
Combative patient				
Checking for patient status				
Acute triage waiting area				
Escorting family members				
Regularly reassesses patients in triage waiting area as deemed necessary by their condition (at least every 2 to 4 hours)				
Aware of COBRA laws regulating ED patient admissions, transfers, and discharges				
Collaborates with secondary "sorter" triage nurse to improve patient care and expedite flow				

Adapted from: Hasbro Children's Hospital, Emergency Dept.; Providence, R.I.

APPENDIX C

THE CHILDREN'S HOSPITAL OF PHILADELPHIA

EMERGENCY DEPARTMENT NURSING TRIAGE / ASSESSMENT

ARRIVAL TIME _____

SORT TIME _____

MED. RECORD # _____

TRIAGE TIME _____

☐ CRITICAL   ☐ ACUTE   ☐ URGENT   ☐ NON URGENT

| ROOM # | TIME IN ROOM: | ID BAND: ☐ | DATE: |

| PATIENT NAME: | AGE |

STATED CHIEF COMPLAINT: _____

PREVIOUS MEDICAL PROBLEMS: _____

ALLERGIES: _____

CURRENT MEDICATIONS: _____

EXPOSURE TO INFECTIOUS DISEASE
☐ YES   ☐ NO

IMMUNIZATIONS UP TO DATE
☐ YES   ☐ NO

DATE OF LAST TETANUS

NURSING ASSESSMENT

WEIGHT	KG	TEMPERATURE	Heart Rate	Resp. Rate	BP
TIME					

TRAUMA SCORE

TIME

GLASGOW COMA SCALE		On Adm	1 Hr p̄ Adm
Eye Opening	Spontaneous	4	4
	To Voice	3	3
	To Pain	2	2
	None	1	1
Verbal Response	Oriented	5	5
	Confused	4	4
	Inappropriate Words	3	3
	Incomprehensible Sounds	2	2
	None	1	1
Motor Response	Obeys Commands	6	6
	Localizes (Pain)	5	5
	Withdraw (Pain)	4	4
	Flexion (Pain)	3	3
	Extension (Pain)	2	2
	None	1	1
TOTAL			
GCS Convert to	14 - 15	5	5
	11 - 13	4	4
	8 - 10	3	3
	5 - 7	2	2
	3 - 4	1	1
Respiratory Rate	10 - 24	4	4
	25 - 35	3	3
	≥ 35	2	2
	≤ 10	1	1
	0	0	0
Respiratory Effort	Normal	1	1
	Shallow	0	0
	Retractive	0	0
Systolic Blood Pressure	≥ 90	4	4
	70 - 90	3	3
	50 - 70	2	2
	≤ 50	1	1
	0	0	0
Capillary Refill	Normal	2	2
	Delayed	1	1
	None	0	0
TOTAL			

OBJECTIVE ASSESSMENT/DESCRIPTION OF INJURY

_____

INITIAL TREATMENT

MEDICATIONS GIVEN: ACETAMINOPHEN

IBUPROFEN _____

NSS DRESSING ☐   SLING ☐   ICE ☐   SPLINT ☐

X-RAY _____ TIME SENT _____ ANATOMY X-RAYED _____

OTHER: _____

SIGNATURES

TRIAGE RN

SORTER RN

MD

TRAUMA SURGEON

NAME: _____

NOTIFICATION TIME: _____

ARRIVAL TIME: _____

NEUROSURGERY

NAME: _____

NOTIFICATION TIME: _____

ARRIVAL TIME: _____

ED 110 REV. 2/95

Figure 3

Triage documentation record.

Modified from The Children's Hospital of Philadelphia, Emergency Department, Philadelphia.

APPENDIX D

Pediatric Triage Fast Track Criteria

HOURS: Monday–Friday, 6–11 PM, Weekends, 1–11 PM

Nonacute patients with the following chief complaints may be triaged to the fast track area:

Infectious Disease

1. Fever in an otherwise well-appearing child
   a) Children >6 months old with fever ≤39.5° C
   b) Children >2 years old with fever <40.5° C
2. Positive cultures
   a) Return for positive throat culture
   b) Return for positive urine culture and is afebrile (>6 months old).
3. Chickenpox uncomplicated by cellulitis, CNS, or respiratory distress
4. Adenitis—first visit
5. Upper respiratory tract infection or cough in children >2 months old
6. Conjunctivitis
7. Stomatitis (without signs or symptoms of dehydration)

ENT

1. Earache
2. Nontraumatic ear drainage
3. Nosebleeds without active bleeding
4. Sore throat (able to open mouth and swallow without difficulty)

Psychiatry

1. Calm, stable psychiatric patients in need of medical examination.

Gastroenterology

1. Vomiting, diarrhea, nausea (without bile in vomitus, without blood in stool or vomitus, without dehydration)
2. Constipation (without vomiting)
3. Colic
4. Abdominal pain (without tenderness, distention, or guarding). Exclude adolescent females with abdominal or flank pain
5. Umbilical granuloma

GU

1. Dysuria or frequency (without fever or suspicion of sexual assault)
2. Hernia: inguinal or umbilical (without vomiting or severe pain)
3. Urethral discharge in adolescent males (without testicular pain)

Dermatology

1. Rashes (nonpetechial), e.g., eczema, impetigo, scabies, insect bites without allergic reaction, diaper rash, chickenpox, and viral rash except measles

Trauma

1. Minor abrasions or contusions (without head injury)
2. Suture removal
3. Minor burn redressing
4. Minor animal or human bites not requiring sutures

Dental

1. Toothache

Note

1. Seek guidance from ED attending M.D. or charge nurse when unsure of triage decision.
2. These criteria should not be viewed as a fixed policy, but should accompany sound clinical nursing judgment and common sense.
3. All referred patients should be seen in ED unless otherwise indicated by ED attending M.D..
4. Diagnosis-requiring procedures are denoted by asterisk. Sending these patients to fast track is volume dependent.

Modified from The Children's Hospital of Philadelphia, Emergency Department, Philadelphia.

APPENDIX E

Consent for Treatment

Involuntary Consent

Involuntary consent refers to the patient who is unable to give consent because of a physical or mental impairment. The source of consent varies among states but is generally in the following order: (1) spouse (legally married), (2) spouse (common law), (3) parent, (4) adult child, (5) adult sibling, (6) adult aunt, uncle, or grandparent, and (7) court system.

Special situations do exist under which involuntary consents are initiated. These might include treatment rendered in an abuse situation, treatment needed for a prisoner, or any consent obtained from the court system.

Minor's Consent
Emancipated Minor

An individual who is considered "emancipated" may give consent for her or his own care. Emancipation is a legal determination wherein a particular minor is given adult rights and responsibilities. These determinations vary among states. The following characteristics have been used to determine emancipation: age, maturity, marital status, degree of self-sufficiency, economic independence, membership in the United States Armed Forces, and general ability to comprehend.

Nonemancipated Minor

A nonemancipated minor is unable to give consent for treatment in most situations. The ability of minors to provide their own consent for treatment varies in each state. Many states do have statutes that allow minors to be treated without parental consent for these conditions: sexually transmitted diseases, pregnancy, child abuse, substance abuse, psychiatric disorders, and those conditions where religious belief might result in the parents' refusal of care.

In summary, the emergency department nurse needs to be familiar with the consent laws in the state in which they practice. Additionally, when obtaining consents at triage, the nurse should know the hospital's policy and procedures in this regard.

APPENDIX F

Situations Reportable to the State

Although the patient has a right to privacy and confidentiality, the health care provider has the professional duty and legal responsibility to report certain situations to the state. Because of individual state regulations, ED staff should be aware of specific laws that require mandatory reporting for the state in which one is practicing.

Some common examples of mandatory reporting include but are not limited to the following:

Mandatory Reportable Situations

- Sexual assault/rape
- Child abuse
- Gunshot wounds, stab wounds, or other injuries resulting from violent attacks
- Homicide or suicide attempts
- Physical assault
- Motor vehicle accidents
- Toxic agent exposures
- Patients dead on arrival
- Communicable diseases (including sexually transmitted diseases)

Failure to report required situations to the state can result in civil as well as criminal liability. It is important, therefore, that both physicians and nurses are aware of their state practice laws and promptly communicate pertinent information to authorities.

Modified from Fleisher G, Ludwig S: *Textbook of pediatric emergency medicine,* ed 3, Baltimore, 1993, Williams & Wilkins; and *Emergency nursing core curriculum,* ed 3, Philadelphia, 1987, Saunders.

Modified from *Triage: meeting the challenge,* Park Ridge, Ill., 1992, Emergency Nurses Association.

APPENDIX G

Toxidromes for Poisonings

SUBSTANCE	EFFECTS	
Anticholinergics (atropine, antidepressants [TCA], phenothiazines, antihistamines)	VS:	Fever, tachycardia, hypertension, cardiac arrhythmias (TCA)
	CNS:	Delirium, psychosis, convulsions, coma
	Eye:	Mydriasis
Amphetamines	VS:	Fever, tachycardia, hypertension
	CNS:	Hyperactive, delirious, tremors, myoclonus, psychosis, convulsions
	Eye:	Mydriasis
	Skin:	Sweaty
Narcotics	VS:	Bradycardia, bradypnea, hypotension, hypothermia
	CNS:	Euphoria leading to coma, hyporeflexia
	Eye:	Pinpoint pupils
Organophosphates (and muscarinic mushroom poisoning)	VS:	Bradycardia, tachypnea (secondary to pulmonary manifestations)
	CNS:	Confusion leading to drowsiness and coma, convulsions, muscle fasciculations, weakness leading to paralysis

Substance	Effects
	Eye: Miosis, blurry vision, lacrimation
	Skin: Sweating
	Odor: Garlic
	Misc: Salivation; bronchorrhea, bronchospasm, and pulmonary edema; urinary frequency and diarrhea
Barbiturates, sedatives/hypnotics	VS: Hypothermia, hypotension, bradypnea
	CNS: Confusion leading to coma, ataxia
	Eye: Nystagmus, miosis or mydriasis
	Skin: Vesicles, bullae
Salicylates	VS: Fever, hyperpnea
	CNS: Lethargy leading to coma
	Odor: Oil of wintergreen (with methyisalicylate)
	Misc: Vomiting
Phenothiazines	VS: Postural hypotension, hypothermia, tachycardia, tachypnea
	CNS: A. Lethargy to coma, tremor, convulsions
	B. Extrapyramidal syndromes:
	Ataxia
	Torticollis
	Back arching
	Oculogyric crisis
	Trismus
	Tongue protusion or heaviness
	Eye: Miosis (majority of cases)
Theophylline	VS: Tachycardia, hypotension, cardiac arrhythmias, tachypnea
	CNS: Agitation, convulsions
	Misc: Vomiting

APPENDIX H

Conversion Tables to International Units

TABLE H-1	Conversion of Pounds to Kilograms for Pediatric Weights*								
Pounds → ↓	0	1	2	3	4	5	6	7	8	9
0	0.00	0.45	0.90	1.36	1.81	2.26	2.72	3.17	3.62	4.08
10	4.53	4.98	5.44	5.89	6.35	6.80	7.35	7.71	8.16	8.61
20	9.07	9.52	9.97	10.43	10.88	11.34	11.79	12.24	12.70	13.15
30	13.60	14.06	14.51	14.96	15.42	15.87	16.32	16.78	17.23	17.69
40	18.14	18.59	19.05	19.50	19.95	20.41	20.86	21.31	21.77	22.22
50	22.68	23.13	23.58	24.04	24.49	24.94	25.40	25.85	26.30	26.76
60	27.21	27.66	28.22	28.57	29.03	29.48	29.93	30.39	30.84	31.29
70	31.75	32.20	32.65	33.11	33.56	34.02	34.47	34.92	35.38	35.83
80	36.28	36.74	37.19	37.64	38.10	38.55	39.00	39.46	39.93	40.37
90	40.82	41.27	41.73	42.18	42.63	43.09	43.54	43.99	44.45	44.90
100	45.36	45.81	46.26	46.72	47.17	47.62	48.08	48.53	48.98	49.44
110	49.89	50.34	50.80	51.25	51.71	52.16	52.61	53.07	53.52	53.97
120	54.43	54.88	55.33	55.79	56.24	56.70	57.15	57.60	58.06	58.51
130	58.96	59.42	59.87	60.32	60.78	61.23	61.68	62.14	62.59	63.05
140	63.50	63.95	64.41	64.86	65.31	65.77	66.22	66.67	67.13	67.58

Pounds →	0	1	2	3	4	5	6	7	8	9
150	68.04	68.49	68.94	69.40	69.85	70.30	70.76	71.21	71.66	72.12
160	72.57	73.02	73.48	73.93	74.39	74.84	75.29	75.75	76.20	76.65
170	77.11	77.56	78.01	78.47	78.92	79.38	79.83	80.28	80.74	81.19
180	81.64	82.10	82.55	83.00	83.46	83.91	84.36	84.82	85.27	85.73
190	86.18	86.68	87.09	87.54	87.99	88.45	88.90	89.35	89.81	90.26
200	90.72	91.17	91.62	92.08	92.53	92.98	93.44	93.89	94.34	94.80

*To obtain kilogram equivalent of 15 pounds, read 10 pounds on side scale, then 5 pounds on top scale. The kilogram equivalent is 6.80.

TABLE H-2   Conversion Factors for Temperature*

CELSIUS	FAHRENHEIT	CELSIUS	FAHRENHEIT	CELSIUS	FAHRENHEIT	CELSIUS	FAHRENHEIT
34.0	93.2	36.4	97.5	38.6	101.5	41.0	105.9
34.2	93.6	36.6	97.9	38.8	101.8	41.2	106.1
34.4	93.9	36.8	98.2	39.0	102.2	41.4	106.5
34.6	94.3	37.0	98.6	39.2	102.6	41.6	106.8
34.8	94.6	37.2	99.0	39.4	102.9	41.8	107.2
35.0	95.0	37.4	99.3	39.6	103.3	42.0	107.6
35.2	95.4	37.6	99.7	39.8	103.6	42.2	108.0
35.4	95.7	37.8	100.0	40.0	104.0	42.4	108.3
35.6	96.1	38.0	100.4	40.2	104.4	42.6	108.7
35.8	96.4	38.2	100.8	40.4	104.7	42.8	109.0
36.0	96.8	38.4	101.1	40.6	105.2	43.0	109.4
36.2	97.2			40.8	105.4		

*(°C) × (9/5) + 32 = °F

(°F − 32) × (5/9) = °C

°C, temperature in Celsius (centigrade) degrees

°F, temperature in Fahrenheit degrees

APPENDIX I

Triage Textbook
Abbreviations

1° & 2° Primary and secondary
ACEP American College of Emergency Physicians
BP Blood pressure
c/o Complaint of . . .
Code "R" Sexual Assault
CVA Costal vertebral angle
DBP Diastolic blood pressure
DIC Disseminated intravascular coagulation
Dx Diagnosis
ED Emergency department
ENA Emergency nurses association
Fx Fracture
GCS Glasgow Coma Scale

HIV Human immunodeficiency virus
HR Heart rate
HRS Hours
HSP Henoch-Schonlein purpura
Hx History
ICP Increased intracranial pressure
ITP Idiopathic thrombocytopenia purpura
JVD Jugular venous distension
NKDA No known drug allergies
NPO Nothing by mouth
NSS Normal sterile saline
ROM Range of motion
RR Respiratory rate

SBP Systolic blood pressure
SCAN Suspected child abuse and neglect
S/P Status post . . .
S_pO_2 Pulse oximetry oxygen saturation
SQ Subcutaneous
Sx Symptom
Sz Seizure
UA Urinalysis
URI Upper respiratory infection
UTI Urinary tract infection
VP Ventriculoperitoneal
Yo Years old
Yrs Years

References

Textbook of pediatric advanced life support, 1994. The American Heart Association:

Resources for optimal care of the injured patient, 1993. American College of Surgeons Committee on Trauma

Barkin R, Rosen P: *Emergency pediatrics: a guide to ambulatory care,* St. Louis, 1991, Mosby.

Budassi Sheehey S: *Emergency nursing principles and practices,* ed 3, St. Louis, 1992, Mosby.

Buschiazzo L: Development or revision of a nurse triage system. In *The handbook of emergency nursing management,* Rockville, Md, 1987, Aspen Publishers.

Emergency Nurses Association: *Emergency nursing core curriculum,* ed 4, Philadelphia, 1994, W.B. Saunders.

Emergency Nurses Association: *Emergency nursing pediatric course (provider) manual,* Chicago, 1993.

Emergency Nurses Association: *Pediatric emergency nursing resource guide,* Chicago, 1993.

Emergency Nurses Association: *Triage: meeting the challenge,* Chicago, 1992.

Emergency Nurses Association: *Emergency nursing care curriculum,* ed 3, Philadelphia, 1987, W.B. Saunders.

Fleisher G, Ludwig S: *Textbook of pediatric emergency medicine,* ed 2, Baltimore, 1988, Williams & Wilkins.

Fleisher G, Ludwig S: *Textbook of pediatric emergency medicine,* ed 3, Baltimore, 1993, Williams & Wilkins.

Frew S: *Patient transfers: how to comply with the law,* Irving, Texas, 1991, American College of Emergency Physicians.

Grossman M, Dieckmann R: *Pediatric emergency medicine,* Philadelphia, 1991, J.B. Lippincott.

Hazinski MF: *Nursing care of the critically ill child,* ed 2, St. Louis, 1992, Mosby.

Henretig F: Toxicologic emergencies. In Fleisher G, Ludwig S: *Textbook of pediatric emergency medicine,* ed 3, Baltimore, 1993, Williams & Wilkins.

Immunization schedule for healthy infants and children, 1995. American Academy of Pediatrics Advisory Committee on Immunization Practices

Memmer M: Acute orthostatic hypotension, *Heart Lung* 17 (2): 134–43, 1988.

Rice M, Abel C: Triage. In Budassi Sheehey S: *Emergency nursing: principles and practices,* ed 3, St. Louis, Mosby.

Seidel HM, Ball JW, Dains JE, Benedict GW: *Mosby's guide to physical examination,* ed 3, St. Louis, 1995, Mosby.

Thibodeau GA, Patton KT: *Anatomy & physiology,* ed 2, St. Louis, 1993, Mosby.

Thomas DO: Pediatric triage and assessment. In Budassi Sheehey S: *Emergency nursing: principles and practice,* ed 3, St. Louis, 1992, Mosby.

Thompson JM: *Mosby's clinical nursing,* ed 3, St. Louis, 1993, Mosby.

Wong DL: *Whaley & Wong's nursing care of infants and children,* ed 5, St. Louis, 1995, Mosby.